PSYCHIATRY - THEORY, APPLICATIONS AND TREATMENTS

ANTIDEPRESSANTS

PHARMACOLOGY, HEALTH EFFECTS AND CONTROVERSY

PSYCHIATRY - THEORY, APPLICATIONS AND TREATMENTS

Additional books in this series can be found on Nova's website under the Series tab.

Additional e-books in this series can be found on Nova's website under the e-books tab.

PHARMACOLOGY - RESEARCH, SAFETY TESTING AND REGULATION

Additional books in this series can be found on Nova's website under the Series tab.

Additional e-books in this series can be found on Nova's website under the e-books tab.

ANTIDEPRESSANTS

PHARMACOLOGY, HEALTH EFFECTS AND CONTROVERSY

LOUIS J. MÍGNE
AND
JASON W. POST
EDITORS

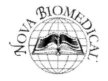

Nova Science Publishers, Inc.
New York

Library of Congress Cataloging-in-Publication Data

ISBN: 978-1-62081-555-7

Library of Congress Control Number: 2012935163

Published by Nova Science Publishers, Inc. † New York

CONTENTS

PREFACE

Antidepressants are the category of drugs that act in a disease specific way to reverse the neuropathological basis of the symptoms of depression. In this book, the authors present current research in the study of the pharmacology, health effects and controversy relating to the use of antidepressants. Topics discussed in this compilation include the biology of fetal exposure to serotonin reuptake inhibitors; the addictive potential of antidepressant drugs; the immunomodulatory action of fluoxetine in normal and in pathological conditions; use of antidepressants in older people with mental illness; and the treatment of comorbid depression and alcohol abuse/dependence with antidepressant medications.

Chapter 1- This chapter will discuss the biology of exposure to antidepressants during pregnancy as it interacts with fetal neurodevelopment. A systematic review of prevalence rates in pregnancy found 12% of women in third trimester meet criteria for depression and the Avon Longitudinal Study of Parents and Children (ALSPAC) found that more women were depressed at 32 weeks pregnant than 8 weeks postpartum. Untreated depression in pregnancy has been associated with increased pregnancy complications, poorer child development and increased risk of postnatal depression. While psychological treatments are indicated for many women with antenatal depression, pharmacological treatment may be indicated for those who either don't respond, have moderate to severe depressive symptoms, or don't have access to psychological treatments. Antidepressants may also be indicated for women with Anxiety Disorders. The most commonly prescribed antidepressants are the selective serotonin reuptake inhibitors (SSRIs). Rates of prescription in North America for antidepressants in pregnancy are rising yet the implications for exposure on the child's longer term neurodevelopment are still relatively unknown. Until now, the limited number of studies has not revealed any effects on global cognitive function. Yet there have been 5 studies published recently which suggest an effect of exposure on psychomotor development and a single, unreplicated study which suggested an increased risk of autism-spectrum disorders in children exposed to these antidepressants in pregnancy.

This chapter includes a brief review of the published research on neuro-developmental outcomes for children following exposure to anti-depressants in pregnancy and in particular, findings on psychomotor development. Methodo-logical limitations in this body of literature including sample size, the measures of child development, the age of the children assessed and potential confounding variables will be discussed.

Several models can be used to understand these findings and the chapter will discuss models such as DOHaD's fetal programming concept and neuro-developmental teratology. While structural teratology is generally limited to the first trimester, neurodevelopmental teratology recognizes the long term effects of exposure to agents or events across pregnancy that can have effect on child development that are often not apparent until well beyond infancy.

In the second half of the chapter, the origins and principles of neuro-developmental teratology are outlined and discussed in the context of the developing serotonin system. This includes an overview of the development and functioning of the serotonin system and the pharmacology of SSRIs in order to consider how these might interact. An overview will be presented of the key animal and human studies on the effects of SSRIs on the developing serotonin system. Finally, implications and suggestions for future research are discussed.

Chapter 2- Antidepressant drugs are relatively efficient psychopharma-cologic agents that are widely used in the treatment of anxiety and affective disorders although controversies are attached to their adverse reactions' profile. In particular, the possibility of this family of drugs to withhold addictive potentials has not been profoundly studied in the literature although it might be encountered in daily clinical practice. In fact, many case reports described antidepressant drug abuse or dependence such as in the case of misuse of antidepressant drugs having amphetamine-like properties. Misuse of antidepressants concern mainly patients with a diagnosis of personality disorder and a previous history of drug or alcohol abuse and who are treated for a depressive disorder. Methadone treated patients are often prone to antidepressant drugs misuse. The latter may enhance the rewarding effect of other psychoactive drugs. From a neurobiological perspective, antidepressant drugs act on the same monoamines involved in addiction. Conversely, the pharmacodynamic profiles of most antidepressants and the absence of acute "desirable" effects in therapeutic dosages make addiction theoretically unlikely. However, rare cases of antidepressant drugs misuse exist in the literature. Discontinuation syndrome and tachyphylaxis/ tolerance are both frequently encountered aspects of antidepressant drugs usage. They correspond to the physical component of the dependence on this class of drugs and are in no means sufficient or indicative of a predisposition or a presence of a dependence on antidepressant drugs. Accordingly, their occurrence should never be confounded with the very rare typical dependence on antidepressant drugs. In this chapter, a review of the literature intends to cover all aspects of this controversial issue regarding antidepressant drugs safety.

Chapter 3- "Antidepressant" is the category of drug that acts in a disease specific way to reverse the neuropathological basis of the symptoms of depression. Symptoms of depression include depressed mood, diminished pleasure, change in appetite or weight, alterations in sleep, psychomotor retardation, fatigue, inability to concentrate, indecisiveness, and thoughts of suicide.

This review aim to show the pharmacology, health effects and controversy related to antidepressants. All currently available antidepressants can be classified into 3 classes: (1) MAOIs, (2) biogenic amine neurotransmitters (3) serotonin type 2A receptor blockers.

Here we considered the antidepressants which are pharmacologically as effective as the WHO claims them to be. Overprescription and misuse of antidepressants is harmful. Over the past decade, the tricyclic antidepressants have been replaced by SSRIs. But it is still controversial whether the newer antidepressants are as effecteive as the older generation compounds. This is also a part of discussion whether antidepressants are helpful in changing the rate of suicide cases and the effect of antidepressants changes with season, nation and gender? Pharmaceutical companies are seeking compounds that can block all the three transporters (the acronym of which is *SNUB* or *super neurotransmitter uptake blocker*). Pharmacogenetics is also helpful treatment of depression. Research has shown that the response to an SSRI is predicted by the genotype of the patient with respect to his or her serotonin transporter.

Chapter 4- Antidepressants are used to alleviate mood disorders, such as major depression, dysthymia and anxiety. Among these drugs, selective serotonin reuptake inhibitors such as fluoxetine, act on neuronal cells by targeting the serotonin transporter prolonging the availability of this neurotransmitter on the synaptic space. In the past years, controversial evidences indicate that antidepressants can modulate non-neuronal cell types. Contradictory data indicate both stimulatory and inhibitory effects of antidepressants in immune cells as well as in tumor cells. First, antidepressants are able to reverse the alterations of the immune system observed in humans suffering depression as well as in animal models of stress. However, fluoxetine also has an effect per se on the immune cells in physiological conditions. Systemic and in vitro fluoxetine administration has been shown to both enhance and inhibit the immune function. The modulatory effect of fluoxetine on the immune function appears to depend on: a) the dose of antidepressant tested and b) the degree of lymphocyte activation. At least in part, this effect is dependent of serotonin reuptake. However, novel pathways that are in part independent of the fluoxetine action on the serotonin transporter are starting to emerge. Interestingly, several antidepressants induce apoptosis in certain kinds of tumors, but also stimulate proliferation on other cancer types. Fluoxetine is one of the most studied antidepressant in this scenario, and was found to affect tumor progression by specific and compensatory mechanisms, some of them seem to be mediated by its action upon the central nervous system, but others are executed directly on peripheral cells.

Chapter 5- *Aims*: The objective of the study was to provide observational clinical data on psychotropic drugs used in older people with mental illness.

Method: This was an observational, single-centre, one-week prevalence study of psychiatric symptoms, disorders and psychotropic/antidepressant drug use in older people with mental illness cared for by the South West people Yorkshire Mental Health NHS Trust (Wakefield Locality), UK. The clinical assessment included completion of the Psychosis Evaluation Tool for Common use by Caregivers.

Results: A total of 593/660 older patients with mental illness (mean±SD age, 76±8.1 years) were assessed). 44.5% had dementia (excluding vascular dementia) and 33.7% had a mood disorder. Of the total, 20.4% did not receive CNS active medication and 46.2% of patients were prescribed an antidepressant. Antidepressants were commonly prescribed where the primary diagnosis was not depression including vascular dementia (31%), dementia (26.1%), schizophrenia and related disorders (26.2%) and anxiety disorders (51.5%). SSRIs were the most commonly prescribed drugs (63.2%) followed by TCAs (22.4%), venlafaxine (9%), mirtazapine (3.2%), reboxetine (1.8%) and phenelzine (0.36%). The single most commonly prescribed drug was paroxetine (n=77) which accounted for 27.7% of all prescriptions. Medications were well tolerated but some patients prescribed a TCA received relatively small doses. Patients with non-vascular dementia received a significantly lower dose of paroxetine compared with other diagnostic groups (F=3.14, p<0.02) though this was still within the recommended/therapeutic range.

Conclusions: Antidepressants are commonly used in older people with mental illness including dementia, schizophrenia and anxiety disorders as well as for patients with a primary diagnosis of depression. Antidepressants are generally well tolerated and patients were broadly satisfied with their medication. The evidence for the use of low dose TCAs in older people remains controversial and further work is needed in this area.

Declaration of interest: None

Chapter 6- Alcohol use disorders are often accompanied by symptoms of other major psychiatric syndromes which may precede, follow, or be concurrent but independent of alcohol misuse. Epidemiological and clinical studies provide evidence that at least two-thirds of alcohol abusing individuals present with clinically significant symptoms of anxiety, sadness, mania-like conditions, other substance use disorders and antisocial behaviours [1, 2, 3, 4]. Affective disorders, including major depression, dysthymia or bipolar disorder, have been shown to be among the most frequent psychiatric disorders that co-occur with alcohol dependence [3, 5, 6, 7]. It is reported that in community samples there is a 2- to 4-fold greater lifetime risk for developing one disorder when the other disorder is present and that this risk is even higher in treatment settings [8]. The co-occurrence of affective and alcohol disorders aggravates the clinical course, treatment outcome, and prognosis for each one of them. Individuals with both disorders have significantly increased rates of alcohol relapse, more severe symptoms, increased suicide risk, poorer treatment compliance and response, severe social and occupational impairment and disability, and consequently higher health services costs [9, 10, 11, 12, 13]. In this context, a growing literature related to the treatment of comorbid depression and alcohol dependence has developed during the last decade, which suggests that antidepressants could be of help in the management of depressed alcoholics.

In: Antidepressants   ISBN: 978-1--62081-555-7
Editors: L. J. Mígne and J. W. Post   © 2012 Nova Science Publishers, Inc.

Chapter 1

THE BIOLOGY OF FETAL EXPOSURE TO SEROTONIN REUPTAKE INHIBITORS: IMPLICATIONS FOR NEURODEVELOPMENT

Megan Galbally[1], Andrew.J. Lewis[2], Salvatore Gentile[3], Susan Walker,[4] and Anne Buist[5]

[1]Mercy Hospital for Women
[2]School of Psychology, Deakin University
[3]Department of Mental Health, ASL Salerno, Italy
[4]Department of Obstetrics and Gynaecology, University of Melbourne
[5]Department of Psychiatry, University of Melbourne

ABSTRACT

This chapter will discuss the biology of exposure to antidepressants during pregnancy as it interacts with fetal neurodevelopment. A systematic review of prevalence rates in pregnancy found 12% of women in third trimester meet criteria for depression and the Avon Longitudinal Study of Parents and Children (ALSPAC) found that more women were depressed at 32 weeks pregnant than 8 weeks postpartum. Untreated depression in pregnancy has been associated with increased pregnancy complications, poorer child development and increased risk of postnatal depression. While psychological treatments are indicated for many women with antenatal depression, pharmacological treatment may be indicated for those who either don't respond, have moderate to severe depressive symptoms, or don't have access to psychological treatments. Antidepressants may also be indicated for women with Anxiety Disorders. The most commonly prescribed antidepressants are the selective serotonin reuptake inhibitors (SSRIs). Rates of prescription in North America for antidepressants in pregnancy are rising yet the implications for exposure on the child's longer term neurodevelopment are still relatively unknown. Until now, the limited number of studies has not revealed any effects on global cognitive function. Yet there have been 5 studies published recently which suggest an effect of exposure on psychomotor development and a single, unreplicated study which suggested an increased risk of autism-spectrum disorders in children exposed to these antidepressants in pregnancy.

This chapter includes a brief review of the published research on neurodevelopmental outcomes for children following exposure to antidepressants in pregnancy and in particular, findings on psychomotor development. Methodological limitations in this body of literature including sample size, the measures of child development, the age of the children assessed and potential confounding variables will be discussed.

Several models can be used to understand these findings and the chapter will discuss models such as DOHaD's fetal programming concept and neurodevelopmental teratology. While structural teratology is generally limited to the first trimester, neurodevelopmental teratology recognizes the long term effects of exposure to agents or events across pregnancy that can have effect on child development that are often not apparent until well beyond infancy.

In the second half of the chapter, the origins and principles of neurodevelopmental teratology are outlined and discussed in the context of the developing serotonin system. This includes an overview of the development and functioning of the serotonin system and the pharmacology of SSRIs in order to consider how these might interact. An overview will be presented of the key animal and human studies on the effects of SSRIs on the developing serotonin system. Finally, implycations and suggestions for future research are discussed.

INTRODUCTION

Studies in North America suggest a recent increase in the prescription of antidepressants to pregnant women and these are the most commonly prescribed psychotropic medication in pregnancy [1-3]. However, many of the risks associated with their prescription in pregnancy are still poorly understood.

The likely reason for increasing use of antidepressants in pregnant women is the recognition of the deleterious effect of untreated maternal mental illness (MMI) on pregnancy and child outcomes. For instance, women who present with mental illnesses during pregnancy, including Major Depression, are at increased risk of pregnancy-related complications. These include prematurity, gestational hypertension and low birth weight [4-7]. Maternal mental illness (MMI) has been identified as a leading indirect cause of maternal mortality in both Australia and the U.K [8, 9].

The reason why untreated MMI results in poorer outcomes for offspring is not fully understood. However, the Developmental Origins of Health and Disease paradigm (DOHaD) suggests that pregnancy and infancy is a critical period of growth and development that has lifelong health implications [10]. Indeed, untreated MMI during in-utero and infant development has been associated with poorer child development, lower IQ, childhood behavioural problems, antisocial tendencies and altered stress regulation as measured by cortisol levels in pre-adolescence [11-13].

While mental illness can be effectively treated with psychological and pharmacological treatments, this review is focused on recent studies examining the use of pharmacological treatment in pregnancy. While one study that examined antidepressant treatment for Major Depression in pregnancy has shown higher risks of relapse when medications are ceased during pregnancy [14], another more recently found no difference in relapse rates whether women ceased or maintained antidepressants [15]. These studies had some significant methodological differences including patient population and severity of illness. In particular severity of illness has been previously associated with efficacy of antidepressants in adult patient populations [16].

While there is increasing information regarding the structural teratological and malformation risk with antidepressant exposure in pregnancy, the information available regarding any longer term neurodevelopmental teratological effect is limited. A systematic review until the end of 2009 identified 12 studies [17] and since then there have been a further 9 studies published.

There have also been several studies which have examined neuro-behavioural effects on fetal and neonatal behaviour and some have postulated this may link to later effects. The observed neonatal neurobehavioural symptoms have been confirmed in a meta-analysis [18] and are predominantly neurological and gastrointestinal symptoms [19]. It has been unclear if these symptoms represent a serotonin discontinuation or toxicity in the neonate. A more recent study has shown that neurobehavioral differences in exposed offspring may be demonstrated from as early as third trimester [20].

However, a recent study by Warburton and Oberlander found there was no difference in neonatal outcomes if antidepressants were stopped 14 days prior to delivery or maintained until delivery [21]. They concluded that their findings suggest a "sustained neurobiological disturbance...rather than an acute pharmacological phenomenon associated with ...withdrawal or acute toxicity" [21]. In addition to poor neonatal adaptation neonates exposed to antidepressants in pregnancy have also been shown to have increased motor activity and lower hear rate variability [22] and reduced pain response [23]. However, a study which followed exposed infants until 8 months of age found no difference in child development between those who were symptomatic and non-symptomatic as neonates [24].

The difficulty in understanding the variation in findings and linking this to underlying mechanisms arises from the methodological limitations of studies available to date. Since ethical considerations limit the capacity of researchers to conduct blinded placebo randomised controlled trials the majority of studies use a case-control prospective cohort design, typically with small numbers and most follow up for less than one year. These studies often suffer from lack of power and possible recruitment bias. Examination of large population based data sets are informative for prescription rates and broad based screening for major developmental deficits, but such population studies tend to lack detail regarding the amount and timing of prenatal exposures and the limitations associated with using brief survey instruments as primary outcome measures. Such deficiencies make it difficult to make any definitive assertions regarding developmental effects from exposure to antidepressants in pregnancy.

SYSTEMATIC LITERATURE REVIEW

Gentile and Galbally conducted in late 2009 a computerized Medline/Pub Med/TOXNET/EMBASE search for the period between January 1973 and December 2009 using the following key-words: pregnancy, child/infant development/neurodevelopment, antidepressants. A separate search was also performed to complete the safety profile of all single medications. Resultant articles were cross-referenced for other relevant articles not identified in the initial search. Extensive manual review of pertinent journals and textbooks was also performed. Searches provided 471 articles, identified on the basis of their abstract or the full-text version when the abstract was unavailable. Only studies reporting primary data on neurocognitive and psychological development of infants exposed in-utero to antidepressants selected and therefore twelve studies met criteria for inclusion. This systematic review has been published in the Journal of Affective Disorders [17].

There were 12 studies identified which met criteria [17]. Of these 12 identified studies only four had studied children to four years or older and only one study had used the Wechsler testing assessments which are regarded as the gold standard of cognitive assessment and have greatest concurrent and predictive validity for assessing child development from four years of age onwards through the life span. The one study which used the Wechsler Preschool and Primary Scale of Intelligence (WPPSI) was published as an abstract and gave little information on potential confounding variables such as maternal depression, other exposures of alcohol, nicotine or illicit substances, and they only examined fluoxetine exposure.

Since this published systematic review was undertaken a further systematic review using the same search strategy has been undertaken to include literature published from December 2009 until December 2011. There have been 9 further studies identified [25-33].

The studies which have examined neurodevelopmental outcomes have predominantly either measured cognitive and motor development or behavioural and child adjustment outcomes. Some studies have measured both.

a. Studies on Cognitive and Motor Development

A prospective, longitudinal study was conducted on two small groups of children exposed to fluoxetine (FLX) either during the first trimester of their intrauterine life or during the entire duration of pregnancy [34]. Both groups were compared with children exposed *in utero* to non-teratogenic agents (such as acetaminophen, penicillin, or dental x-ray films). There were no differences in IQ values and neurobehavioural performances between the groups.

Concordant results emerged from a study which evaluated cognitive and language development and behavior in children exposed *in utero* to either tricyclic antidepressants (TCAs) or FLX. Three groups of mother-child pairs were recruited: two groups included women counseled during the first trimester of pregnancy because they had needed antidepressant medications [35]. A control group exposed to non-teratogenic agents was also engaged. The mean global IQ values were similar between the groups, as well as scores on language performance tests. Moreover, the groups failed to demonstrate any differences in temperament, mood, arousability, reactivity, activity level, distractibility, and behavior problems. The study did not specify maternal daily dosage of antidepressants, but- importantly- potential confounding variables (such as degree of maternal depression, maternal IQ, and socio-economic status) were controlled for.

Two more recent studies, both published as abstracts, also found no signs of neurodevelopmental teratogenicity in infants whose mothers had been treated with either selective serotonin reuptake inhibitors (SSRIs) or specifically, FLX [36, 37].

A further prospective, controlled study investigated children exposed *in utero* to wide ranges of maternal FLX daily dose because their mothers were diagnosed with major unipolar depression and were found to require pharmacotherapy [38]. This group was matched with two groups: one exposed to TCAs and a control which was unexposed to medications. The study failed to demonstrate any unwanted consequence of TCA or FLX exposure on cognitive, language, and behavioral development. Nevertheless, eventual relationships between maternal daily dosages of FLX and quality of children's performances in neurodevelopmental tests were not investigated, whereas the following factors were entered as independent variables: mother's IQ and socio-economic status, ethanol and nicotine use, duration and severity of depression, number of depressive episodes after delivery, and medications used for depression treatment.

There is a limited amount of literature examining children exposed to psychotropic drugs throughout both pregnancy and lactation [39]. In this case, mothers had been treated with citalopram (CIT) without any apparent detrimental effect on the main neurodevelopmental milestones as clinically assessed by a pediatrician and physiotherapist.

To compare the structural growth and developmental outcome of children born to mothers who were exposed or not exposed to SSRIs *in utero*, Casper and colleagues recruited a small number children of depressed mothers treated with SSRIs during pregnancy, and compared on birth outcomes and post-natal neurodevelopmental functioning with children whose mothers were diagnosed with major depressive disorder in pregnancy, and elected not to take medications [40]. Prenatal SSRI exposure seemed to be associated with subtle adverse effects on both motor development and motor control: these effects were consistent with the pharmacologic properties of the drugs [41]. Drug-exposed children were rated significantly lower than unexposed children on psychomotor development indexes.

Although, the children's mental development and their attention, orientation, and emotional regulation were analogous in both groups. The differences were particularly notable for tremulousness and for fine motor movements both of which showed a moderate to large effect size with a Cohen's d=0.60 and 0.94 respectively. However, the major limitations of this study to be highlighted include the small sample size which meant the four antidepressants were grouped together for analysis (versus analyzing each antidepressant separately), and alcohol usage was significantly more frequent in the exposed group.

In a case control study , 435 mother-infant pairs who had redeemed a prescription for psychoactive drugs during pregnancy were followed up [42]. In this group, the largest number of women was treated with antidepressant agents. As controls, children of women who had not redeemed any prescriptions of psychotropic or anti-epileptic drug during pregnancy were randomly selected. All the children were examined by specific psychomotor development test: the BOEL. Among 340 children with maternal exposure to benzodiazepines, antidepressants, neuroleptics, and anti-epileptics during pregnancy, the test was abnormal in 53 (16%). Among the controls, the test was abnormal in 4% of children, even after appropriate adjusting for confounding variables. The crude odds ratio for abnormal test in children exposed to antidepressant medications was 4.5.

More recently, a study of 22 children exposed and 19 controls prospectively followed since pregnancy found a moderate effect size for fine motor (Cohen's d=0.47) and gross motor (Cohen's d=.43) on the Bayley's Scales of Infant Development [25]. These children were tested between 18-35 months of age [25]. These findings did not reach statistical significance due to lack of power. This study found no difference between the groups on total score on the BSID.

The detrimental effects of prenatal exposure to antidepressants on psychomotor performance may also depend on the length/duration of exposure with Casper et al. finding longer duration of exposure to antidepressants in pregnancy associated with lower Psychomotor Developmental Index score at 14 months of age [28].

A study from the Danish National Cohort found that children exposed to antidepressants in pregnancy had poorer motor development at 6 months of age but this was not found at 19 months of age [32].

Oberlander et al. compared neonatal and infantile behavior following intrauterine exposure (during both second and third trimester of gestation) to single-agent SSRIs (group 1) or SSRIs plus clonazepam (group 2) [24]. The control group consisted of 23 unexposed infants. Although signs of poor neonatal adaptation were demonstrated in nearly 30% of SSRI exposed infants, later developmental outcome was normal, without differences between infants affected by neonatal adverse reactions and asymptomatic infants.

A recent study which examined early infant neurobehavioral development, (as measured by the Brazelton Neonatal Behavioral Assessment Scale), at 1 week and then 6-8 weeks of age found no difference in infants exposed to antidepressants compared to controls [29].

In contrast, a number of studies [19, 22] and a meta-analysis [18] have found exposure to antidepressants is associated with altered neurobehaviour in neonates. A recent study which utilized the NICU Network Neurobehavioural Scale, a validated scale specifically designed to assess neurological and behavioural function of infants exposed to drugs, found SSRI exposed neonates had more startles, tremor and hypertonic reflexes than non-exposed controls or among infants with depressed mothers not receiving antidepressant treatment [30].

In addition, recent evidence seems to suggest that neonates who develop neurobehavioral symptoms as a consequence of intrauterine exposure to antidepressants are at increased risk for social-behavioural abnormalities on the Denver Developmental Test at 2-6 years of age [31].

b. Studies on Child Adjustment and Emotional Development

Nulman et al [38] and Morison et al [36], in addition to examining child neurocognitive development both also examined infant/toddler temperament and Morison also examined parent-child relations. Both studies found no differences between exposed and control groups on these measures.

Two further, interesting studies performed by the same group of researchers also provided reassuring findings about the long-term behavioral outcome of infants exposed *in utero* to SSRIs. The first of these studies actually concluded that the main clinical features characterizing impaired internalizing behaviors (such as emotional hyper-reactivity, anxiety, depression, irritability, and withdrawal) were not affected by prenatal exposure to antidepressant medications [43].

Symptoms associated with poor externalizing behaviors (including noncompliance, verbal/physical aggression, disruptive acts, and emotional outbursts) were also found to be unaffected by maternal SSRI treatment during pregnancy [44].

However, a more recent study by Oberander et al. found antenatal exposure to SSRIs was associated with an increased risk of internalizing disorders as measured by the Child Behaviour Checklist (CBCL) even after controlling for pre and post partum maternal anxiety (F=3.978, P=.05, η^2=0.06) [45].

c. Studies on the Quality of Parent-Child Relationship

Reebye et al examined both neurocognitive development using the Bayley Scales of Infant Development (BSID) at 2 months of age and parent-child relations using the Parent-Child Early Relational Assessment Scale (PC-ERAS) and found no difference between study and exposed groups on either measure [46].

d. Studies on the Risk of Specific Disorders

Figueroa examined claims-based data in the U.S. for attention deficit disorder (ADHD) in children who had been exposed to antidepressants in pregnancy [26]. This study found that prenatal exposure to bupropion might increase the risk of developing ADHD, but exposure to SSRIs did not show any increase in this risk.

Croen et al in a population based case-control study found a potential relationship between antenatal exposure to antidepressant medications and Autism Spectrum Disorder (ASD), since 20 of 298 (6.7%) children diagnosed with (ASD) were found to be exposed in utero to such drugs, compared to 3.3% of controls. The limitations of this study include lack of independent verification of diagnosis of ASD and exposure was based on a prescription having been filled. Hence, in their article Croen et al. state by cautioning that "it is reasonable to conclude that prenatal SSRI exposure is very unlikely to be a major risk factor for ASD"[47]. Moreover, until now these findings have not been replicated and several large population based studies and meta-analyses suggest the lack of specific perinatal risk factors and/or single causes for ASD [48, 49].

THE BIOLOGY OF EXPOSURE

Serotonin System

Serotonergic neurons evolved around 500 million years ago together with fundamental structures in the vertebrate brain. Serotonin- named in 1947 after the discovery of its ability to constrict blood vessels- has a wide influence across several regulatory mechanisms including mood, appetite, thermo-regulation, sleep-wake, sexual behaviours, motor and pain perception [50, 51]. In addition, the neurotransmitter serotonin regulates the development of key neural tissues such as the hippocampus and somatosensory cortex [52], and mediates the positive outgrowth and survival of neurons [53]. Serotonin also modulates the response of neurons to other neurotransmitters [54].

The cell bodies of the serotonergic neurons are located around the midline raphe nuclei within the brainstem [55]. However, these cells have projections throughout the brain and spinal cord. Serotonin is found in cells outside the CNS such as platelet and mast cells although it does not cross the blood brain barrier [56]. There are at least 14 different serotonin receptors in the periphery and CNS and serotonin receptors are activated by serotonin and in turn modulate a number of other neurotransmitters and hormones.

The neurotransmitter serotonin is classified as a biogenic amine and it is derived from an amino acid tryptophan [55] which is mostly obtained through dietary sources [56]. Two enzymes are required to synthesize serotonin are tryptophan hydroxylase and 5-hydroxytryptophan decarboxylase and degradation of serotonin is caused by monoamine oxidase.

In classic studies of felines, Jacobs found that serotonergic neurons are involved in the state of arousal in animals - neuronal firing declines with decreasing arousal and increases with waking- stopping entirely with REM sleep and complete muscle inactivity- suggesting the S neurons are involved in the command for muscle activity [54].

Embryology and Serotonin System

The development of the central nervous systems involves processes which include cell proliferation, migration, differentiation, synaptogenesis, myelination and apoptosis [57]. Molecular signals are crucial in this process and neural development requires availability of molecular signals and also the ability of cells to respond to these signals [58].

Serotonergic neurons develop by the 5th week post conception in the developing human brain making it one of the earliest to develop [58]. In the developing brain, serotonin acts as both a neurotransmitter and a molecular signal for neuronal cell growth and differentiation [52, 53, 59, 60]. In particular, it regulates development of the hippocampus and somatosensory cortex [53]. Serotonin controls the development of the serotonergic system [53] and therefore, alterations in serotonin levels also have the potential to impact on the development of the serotonergic system. For example, it is thought that the reduction in serotonin levels as a result of alcohol abuse in pregnancy may occur through a mechanism related to the developing serotonergic system and as a molecular signal may cause some of the wide ranging neurological deficits associated with Fetal Alcohol Syndrome [59].

Two animal models have been used to demonstrate possible effects of increased serotonin on the developing brain, the first is serotonin transporter (SERT) knockout mice and the second is monoamine oxidase (MAO) knockout mice [61]. Both models show altered neuronal development and increased serotonin levels [61]. In following these mice across later development they go on to show changes in behaviour including altered sleep patterns, depression like behaviours and decreased performance on tasks. These findings are in contrast to mice exposed to SSRIs as adults where these effects are not observed. These findings suggest there are different effects of high serotonin levels on the nervous system when exposure occurs in the developing brain than in the adult brain [61].

The Serotonergic system also influences, and is influenced by, the development of the hypothalamic-pituitary-adrenal (HPA) axis. For instance, glucocoticoids can alter serotonin levels and in rat studies have been shown to alter SERT expression and can alter the serotonergic system [62]. Serotonin has been found to alter programming of HPA function during specific periods of development. For instance, serotonin has been found to increase hippo-campal glucocorticoid receptor (GR) mRNA levels in guinea pigs from day 40-50 of gestation [62].

PHARMACOLOGY OF ANTIDEPRESSANTS AND PREGNANCY

To assess the safety of antidepressants in pregnancy the two questions that must be asked are: how much medication is the fetus and infant exposed to, and what effect does this exposure have on fetal, infant and child development. The quantity of medication the fetus and infant is exposed to can be measured in placental passage in utero, and breast milk excretion in the postpartum period. Placental passage studies for the SSRIs have shown variable concentrations although all were much lower than maternal doses [63]. However the concentration did vary between different medications with one study showing sertraline being lower than fluoxetine and it has been noted that there is also individual variability in cord to maternal drug concentration ratios [64].

Therefore, all antidepressants cross the placenta and are excreted in breast milk reaching the infant at 1-10% of the maternal dose. The fetus and infant may be exposed to these medications during several sensitive periods of neurological development although it remains unclear if the level of exposure accompanying treatment with anti-depressants is sufficient to affect child development. A study of timing of exposure to antidepressants in pregnancy found duration of exposure rather than timing was more critical for effects on infant outcomes [65]. Several studies have found a dose effect for exposure to antidepressants in pregnancy and fetal or infant outcomes [19, 66, 67].

DEVELOPMENTAL TERATOLOGY AND SSRIS

The recognition that exposures during pregnancy could increase the risk of malformations is a relatively recent development. Initially, observation focused principally on the effects of exposure in first trimester increasing the risk of an infant being born with structural abnormalities [68, 69]. The most well known is thalidomide, a drug prescribed to pregnant women in the 1950s to treat morning sickness in first trimester and which was observed to result in an increased rate of offspring being born with missing and deformed limbs.

However, the concept of neurodevelopmental teratology has developed in response to observed phenomenon that exposure to some agents such as medications or substances of abuse in pregnancy can result in longer term deficits such as cognitive, behavioural or other functional impairments even in absence of detectable structural anomalies of the central nervous system [68, 69].

When studying the teratogenic potential of any medications, timing of exposure is important given there are "differing windows of vulnerability in the developing fetus."[68,69] However, while structural abnormities are typically associated with early pregnancy exposure, detrimental effects on neurobehavior, motor and cognitive development are potentially associated also with exposure throughout or later in pregnancy [68]. Understanding the potential theoretical mechanism of teratogenic effect is essential in designing studies to examine for potential neurodevelopmental teratogenic effects with in-utero exposure [68].

The serotonin system exercises a regulatory function on muscle tone and motor output which may indicate that the developing motor system is vulnerable to SSRI exposure. In addition, alteration in serotonin levels may have wider neurological developmental effects through its action as a molecular signal for neuronal growth and differentiation.

Studies which have examined the effects of SSRI exposure on neural development have predominantly been undertaken in animal models. This has some inherent flaws given the variation in gestational development and length in many animals. For instance, rats and mice have neural development in the postpartum which is analogous to that of human fetal development [53]. In addition many of the preclinical studies of the effects of in utero exposure to SSRIs were carried out in healthy animals whereas treatment with SSRIs in the clinical setting is with women who are suffering from mental illness and often other co-morbid adversities [53]. Interestingly, a study in rats showed that fluoxetine exposure in the presence of maternal stress protected against a decrease in cell proliferation and neurogenesis in the hippocampus [70]. However, given the significant differences in development, many of the animal studies and modelling are difficult to translate into risks for human offspring.

Those studies which have examined the effects of SSRI and tricyclic antidepressant exposure on neural development in animal models have found exposure does interact with the development of the serotonergic system and through this has effects on the wider neurological development [53]. For instance, a study of fluoxetine in mice found it increased cell proliferation and also had sex-specific effects on neural development [71]. In a study of rats followed until adolescence, fluoxetine exposure altered the neuronal structure and later the functioning of the somatosensory system [72]. Interestingly a study which examined the effects of fluoxetine and imipramine on neuronal growth in the frontal lobe found a decrease in number of neurons from fluoxetine exposure but a more marked decrease with imipramine exposure on the frontal lobe [73]. Despite these findings a study which followed rats to adulthood found no effect of exposure to fluoxetine on developmental outcomes [74] and two studies have found fluoxetine is protective to neural development [70, 75].

To further elucidate any potential effect of SSRIs on neuronal development two markers; S100B and Brain-Derived Neurotrophic Factor

(BDNF), have been studied [53]. Both S100B and BDNF are found centrally and peripherally. S100B is a mediator in neuronal development, in particular neuronal outgrowth and glial cell proliferation [76]. A study in humans has found neonates exposed in pregnancy to SSRIs had significantly lower levels of S100B than neonates not exposed [76]. However, a genetics study which examined methylation of BDNF promoter in neonates exposed in pregnancy to SSRI found no difference in these infants compared to unexposed [77]. This study did find that infants of pregnant women with depressed mood in 2nd trimester had lower SLC6A4 methylation status [77]. SLC6A4 encodes transmembrane serotonin transporter which regulates serotonin reuptake and therefore serotonin levels [77]. This suggests one possible epigenetic mechanism explaining the proposed effect of maternal mood in pregnancy on infant and child outcomes.

There have been some human and animal studies which have shown SSRI exposure in pregnancy may specifically affect motor development [25, 28, 40, 42, 78]. Animal studies have also shown that postnatal rat fluoxetine exposure altered cerebellum development through the activation of 5HT1A receptors [79]. A study of rats exposed to fluoxetine found a delay in motor development [78] and another found reduced locomotor activity in the context of an altered structure of the somatosensory cortex [72]. Interestingly neurobehavioural changes have been shown in humans exposed in utero to SSRIs from third trimester through to infancy [19, 67]. In a study of human neonates exposed to SSRIs in pregnancy the neonatal serotonergic nervous system symptoms were related to cord blood 5-hydroxyindolacetic (5-HIAA) levels [80]. Interestingly, Oberlander et al., found that neonatal outcomes for exposed infants were moderated by polymorphisms of the serotonin transporter promoter geneotype (SLC6A4) [81].

Effects of exposure to SSRIs in pregnancy on the development and function of the peripheral serotonin system have also been examined. Both platelet and neuronal serotonin transporters are encoded by the same gene [82]. A study which examined levels of platelet 5HT levels found these to be significantly lower in neonates exposed in utero to SSRIs [82]. However, a study of breastfeeding found no change in infant platelet 5HT in infants breastfed by mothers taking fluoxetine [83].

In animals, more than a few studies have suggested behavioural or biochemical changes after in utero exposure to antidepressants which act on the serotoninergic system. A study in mice exposed to fluoxetine at the equivalent in human development of third trimester pregnancy showed abnormal emotional behaviour once adults [84] and a further study in mice exposed to fluoxetine also confirmed ongoing changes in behaviour including depressive like symptoms [85]. Furthermore, exposure of mouse embryonic stem cells to fluoxetine has also been shown to increase the differentiation into glial cells suggesting fetal neural development is sensitive to fluoxetine exposure in mice [86]. In studies on rats exposed to citalopram it has been demonstrated that neonatal exposure resulted in lower levels of tryptophan hydroxylase [87] and lower levels of innervations of the hippocampal areas which was also found to be dose dependent [88]. A study of rats exposed to fluoxetine in pregnancy found increased anxiety behaviours as adults [89].

Alterations in both pain and thermal perception have also been found in a number of animal studies and in a single study of human infants [23, 72, 90]. For instance, a study of guinea pigs exposed to fluoxetine showed persistent increase in pain threshold into adulthood [90] as did a study of rats exposed to fluoxetine [72]. The single study of human infants examined pain reactivity in the newborn and then at 2 months of age. Their findings suggested a significant difference in exposed infants for pain reactivity as a newborn and this difference remained at 2 months of age [23].

DEVELOPMENT ORIGINS OF HEALTH AND DISEASE, MATERNAL DEPRESSION AND SSRIS

When balancing any potential risks of medication exposure in pregnancy, including that of neurodevelopmental teratology, these risks must be weighed against emerging evidence for the risk to offspring of exposure to untreated maternal mental illness.

The idea that there are fetal origins for adult disease also termed 'fetal programming' arose from the observation by Barker et al. that low birth weight increased the risk of later cardiovascular disease and type 2 diabetes [91]. However, more recent research has suggested that health may be influenced by a range of factors operating from prior to conception, across pregnancy, and into the postpartum period. Hence the name 'Developmental Origins of Health and Disease (DOHaD)' [91]. DOHaD suggests that the genotype is only one level of inheritance and that phenotype can be influenced by environmental factors, interacting with developmental processes across early life from pre-conception to postpartum [91]. Gene expression is regulated by epigenetic processes that form a complex regulatory system which can activate, silence or alter the transcription of genes [92]. Such processes drive fetal development and are particularly active in neuro-development- suggesting that in utero brain development may be highly attuned to input from the maternal environment.

The DOHaD model suggests that high sensitivity to early environment may shape development in a manner likely to be adaptive in the organism's future- enhancing its fit with the post-natal environment and increasing its chances of survival and ultimately reproduction. This programming function of early development occurs in the form of cell differentiation, growth and homeostatic control shaping development and phenotypic outcome [91]. The health implications of this model arise from the potential for a mis-match between the environment that is predicted by the fetus through cues from mother and placenta, and the actual conditions experienced postnatally [91].

A relevant example is Glover's work on the effects of maternal anxiety and stress in pregnancy which appears to have an impact on fetal development and subsequent child outcomes. In examining the results of the Avon Longitudinal Study of Parents and Children (ALSPAC), a longitudinal, prospective study of women and their children, an association between exposure to maternal anxiety in pregnancy predicted emotional and behavioural problems in four year old children after controlling for postnatal stressors [11].

These findings are consistent with those from a review of 14 prospective studies examining the effects of antenatal maternal anxiety on offspring outcomes, and found effects in poorer emotional regulation from infancy to adolescence [93]. Within the review the authors proposed two potential mechanisms for an association between maternal anxiety and stress in pregnancy and subsequent poorer behavioural, cognitive and emotional outcomes in offspring. The first possible mechanism suggests this association is the result of fetal exposure to high levels of maternal glucocoticoids which cross the placenta resulting in higher fetal cortisol which may impact on neurodevelopment The second proposed mechanism is that maternal anxiety and stress may restrict uterine artery blood flow resulting in a higher resistance index and hence poorer obstetric environment and thus affecting fetal development [93].

One of the difficulties with the first hypothesis is that usually the placenta acts as a barrier protecting the fetus from maternal cortisol through the enzyme, 11ß-hydroxysteroid dehydrogenase type 2 enzyme (11 ß-HSD2) , which acts to metabolise maternal cortisol into inactive products [93]. However, a recent study has found that maternal state and trait anxiety can down regulate placental 11 ß-HSD2 [94]. It has also been suggested that maternal anxiety may permanently alter fetal HPA axis functioning however a recent review did not find strong evidence for this theory [95].

There are some important common principles between DOHaD research and research on the neurodevelopmental effects of in utero exposure to medication. One concerns careful consideration of the timing of exposure within pregnancy in relation to the relevant stage of fetal development. Medication exposure at different stages of pregnancy interacts with different stages of maternal depression. O'Connor et al found exposure to maternal anxiety at 32 weeks associated with poorer outcomes for boys than exposure earlier in pregnancy including hyperactive and emotional problems [11]. However, the findings for timing have not been consistent across both DOHaD and medication exposure studies [93]. Studies which have examined for effects of the offspring's gender have found boys may be more susceptible to exposure to maternal anxiety and stress in pregnancy [93].

Our understanding of how and why maternal mental illness, such as anxiety, may effect fetal and child development is still limited. The extent to which exposures to maternal stress, anxiety and depression- as studies in the DOHaD model- can be used as a model to also understand fetal exposure to anti-depressant medication is a matter for careful consideration. Needless to say, mothers taking antidepressants also expose their infants to any depression or anxiety which might remain untreated by medication. In balancing the risks of treating women with anxiety and depression in pregnancy with anti-depressant medication it will be important to be able to also present a coherent understanding of the risks for offspring of untreated mental illness as well as medication.

CONCLUSION

While there are extensive animal studies and more limited human studies which have examined the effects of antidepressant exposure in utero on offspring development there is as yet no clarity about risks. Future studies in humans are required which follow offspring to later stages of development where outcomes can be more accurately measured. Studies also need to have adequate numbers of participants and controls, adjust for relevant confounders, attempt to separate the effect of illness severity versus teratogenicity of treatment and use adequate neurodevelopmental measures to ensure findings are robust. Current clinical practice suggests a careful individual discussion with women on the risks and benefits to both her and her unborn child when antidepressant treatment is required in pregnancy.

REFERENCES

[1]   Alwan S, Reefhuis J, Rasmussen SA, Friedman JM. Patterns of antidepressant medication use among pregnant women in a United States population. *J. Clin. Pharmacol.* 2011 Feb;51(2):264-70.

[2]   Cooper WO, Willy ME, Pont SJ, Ray WA. Increasing use of antidepressants in pregnancy. *Am. J. Obstet. Gynecol.* 2007 Jun; 196(6):544 e1-5.

[3]   Andrade SE, Raebel MA, Brown J, Lane K, Livingston J, Boudreau D, et al. Use of antidepressant medications during pregnancy: a multisite study. *Am. J. Obstet. Gynecol.* 2008 Feb;198(2):194 e1-5.

[4]   Kurki T, Hiilesmaa V, Raitasalo R, Mattila H, Ylikorkala O. Depression and anxiety in early pregnancy and risk for preeclampsia. *Obstet. Gynecol.* 2000 Apr;95(4):487-90.

[5]   Bonari L, Bennett H, Einarson A, Koren G. Risks of untreated depression during pregnancy. *Can. Fam. Physician* 2004 Jan;50:37-9.

[6]   Bansil P, Kuklina EV, Meikle SF, Posner SF, Kourtis AP, Ellington SR, et al. Maternal and fetal outcomes among women with depression. *J. Womens Health* (Larchmt) Feb;19(2):329-34.

[7]   Jablensky AV, Morgan V, Zubrick SR, Bower C, Yellachich LA. Pregnancy, delivery, and neonatal complications in a population cohort of women with schizophrenia and major affective disorders. *Am. J. Psychiatry* 2005 Jan;162(1):79-91.

[8]   Austin MP, Kildea S, Sullivan E. Maternal mortality and psychiatric morbidity in the perinatal period: challenges and opportunities for prevention in the Australian setting. *Med. J. Aust.* 2007 Apr 2;186(7):364-7.

[9]   Brettingham M. Depression and obesity are major causes of maternal death in Britain. *BMJ* 2004 Nov 20;329(7476):1205.

[10]   Gluckman PD, Hanson MA, Cooper C, Thornburg KL. Effect of in utero and early-life conditions on adult health and disease. *N. Engl. J. Med.* 2008 Jul 3;359(1):61-73.

[11]   O'Connor TG, Heron J, Glover V. Antenatal anxiety predicts child behavioral/emotional problems independently of postnatal depression. *J. Am. Acad. Child Adolesc. Psychiatry* 2002 Dec;41(12):1470-7.

[12] Hay DF, Pawlby S, Waters CS, Sharp D. Antepartum and postpartum exposure to maternal depression: different effects on different adolescent outcomes. *J. Child Psychol. Psychiatry* 2008 Oct;49(10):1079-88.

[13] Deave T, Heron J, Evans J, Emond A. The impact of maternal depression in pregnancy on early child development. *BJOG* 2008 Jul;115(8):1043-51.

[14] Cohen LS, Altshuler LL, Harlow BL, Nonacs R, Newport DJ, Viguera AC, et al. Relapse of major depression during pregnancy in women who maintain or discontinue antidepressant treatment. *JAMA* 2006 Feb 1;295(5):499-507.

[15] Yonkers KA, Gotman N, Smith MV, Forray A, Belanger K, Brunetto WL, et al. Does antidepressant use attenuate the risk of a major depressive episode in pregnancy? *Epidemiology* 2011 Nov;22(6):848-54.

[16] Fournier JC, DeRubeis RJ, Hollon SD, Dimidjian S, Amsterdam JD, Shelton RC, et al. Antidepressant drug effects and depression severity. JAMA: *The Journal of the American Medical Association* 2010; 303(1):47.

[17] Gentile S, Galbally M. Prenatal exposure to antidepressant medications and neurodevelopmental outcomes: a systematic review. *J. Affect Disord* 2010 Jan;128(1-2):1-9.

[18] Lattimore KA, Donn SM, Kaciroti N, Kemper AR, Neal CR, Jr., Vazquez DM. Selective serotonin reuptake inhibitor (SSRI) use during pregnancy and effects on the fetus and newborn: a meta-analysis. *J. Perinatol.* 2005 Sep;25(9):595-604.

[19] Galbally M, Lewis AJ, Lum J, Buist A. Serotonin discontinuation syndrome following in utero exposure to antidepressant medication: prospective controlled study. *Aust. N. Z. J. Psychiatry* 2009 Sep;43(9):846-54.

[20] Mulder EJH, Ververs FFT, de Heus R, Visser GHA. Selective serotonin reuptake inhibitors affect neurobehavioral development in the human fetus. *Neuropsychopharmacology*; 36(10):1961-71.

[21] Warburton W, Hertzman C, Oberlander TF. A register study of the impact of stopping third trimester selective serotonin reuptake inhibitor exposure on neonatal health. *Acta Psychiatr. Scand.* 2010 Jun;121(6):471-9.

[22] Zeskind PS, Stephens LE. Maternal selective serotonin reuptake inhibitor use during pregnancy and newborn neurobehavior. *Pediatrics* 2004 Feb;113(2):368-75.

[23] Oberlander TF, Grunau RE, Fitzgerald C, Papsdorf M, Rurak D, Riggs W. Pain reactivity in 2-month-old infants after prenatal and postnatal serotonin reuptake inhibitor medication exposure. *Pediatrics* 2005 Feb;115(2):411-25.

[24] Oberlander TF, Misri S, Fitzgerald CE, Kostaras X, Rurak D, Riggs W. Pharmacologic factors associated with transient neonatal symptoms following prenatal psychotropic medication exposure. *J. Clin. Psychiatry* 2004 Feb;65(2):230-7.

[25] Galbally M, Lewis AJ, Buist A. Developmental outcomes of children exposed to antidepressants in pregnancy. *Aust. N. Z. J. Psychiatry* 2011 May;45(5):393-9.

[26] Figueroa R. Use of antidepressants during pregnancy and risk of attention-deficit/hyperactivity disorder in the offspring. *J. Dev. Behav. Pediatr* 2010 Oct;31(8):641-8.

[27] Croen LA, Grether JK, Yoshida CK, Odouli R, Hendrick V. Antidepressant use during pregnancy and childhood autism spectrum disorders. *Arch. Gen. Psychiatry* Nov;68(11):1104-12.

[28] Casper RC, Gilles AA, Fleisher BE, Baran J, Enns G, Lazzeroni LC. Length of prenatal exposure to selective serotonin reuptake inhibitor (SSRI) antidepressants: effects on neonatal adaptation and psychomotor development. *Psychopharmacology* 2011:1-9.

[29] Suri R, Hellemann G, Stowe ZN, Cohen LS, Aquino A, Altushuler LL. A Prospective, Naturalistic, Blinded Study of Early Neurobehavioral Outcomes for Infants Following Prenatal Antidepressant Exposure. *The Journal of clinical psychiatry* 2011;72(7):1002-7.

[30] Salisbury AL, Wisner KL, Pearlstein T, Battle CL, Stroud L, Lester BM. Newborn neurobehavioral patterns are differentially related to prenatal maternal major depressive disorder and serotonin reuptake inhibitor treatment. *Depression and Anxiety* 2011.

[31] Klinger G, Frankenthal D, Merlob P, Diamond G, Sirota L, Levinson-Castiel R, et al. Long-term outcome following selective serotonin reuptake inhibitor induced neonatal abstinence syndrome. *Journal of Perinatology* 2011;31(9):615-20.

[32] Pedersen LH, Henriksen TB, Olsen J. Fetal exposure to antidepressants and normal milestone development at 6 and 19 months of age. *Pediatrics* 2011:peds. 2008-3655v1.

[33] Oberlander TF, Papsdorf M, Brain UM, Misri S, Ross C, Grunau RE. Prenatal effects of selective serotonin reuptake inhibitor antidepressants, serotonin transporter promoter genotype (SLC6A4), and maternal mood

on child behavior at 3 years of age. *Arch. Pediatr. Adolesc. Med.* May;164(5):444-51.

[34] Nulman I, Koren G. The safety of fluoxetine during pregnancy and lactation. *Teratology*1996 May;53(5):304-8.

[35] Koren G, Nulman I, Addis A. Outcome of children exposed in utero to fluoxetine: a critical review. *Depress Anxiety* 1998;8 Suppl 1:27-31.

[36] Morison SJ, Grunau RE, Oberlander TF, Misri S, Pannikar H, Reebye P. Infant social behaviour and development in the first year of life following prolonged prenatal psychotropic medication exposure [Abstract]. *Pediatric Research* 2001;49(4 Pt2 Suppl):28A.

[37] Mattson S, Eastvold A, Jones K, Harris J, C. C. Neurobehavioral follow-up of children prenatally exposed to fluoxetine [Abstract]. *Teratology* 1999;59:376.

[38] Nulman I, Rovet J, Stewart DE, Wolpin J, Pace-Asciak P, Shuhaiber S, et al. Child development following exposure to tricyclic antidepressants or fluoxetine throughout fetal life: a prospective, controlled study. *Am J Psychiatry* 2002 Nov;159(11):1889-95.

[39] Hekkinen T, Ekblad U, Kero P, Ekblad S, Laine K. Citalopram in pregnancy and lactation. *Clinical Pharmacology Therapeutics* 2002;72(2):184-91.

[40] Casper RC, Fleisher BE, Lee-Ancajas JC, Gilles A, Gaylor E, DeBattista A, et al. Follow-up of children of depressed mothers exposed or not exposed to antidepressant drugs during pregnancy. *J. Pediatr.* 2003 Apr;142(4):402-8.

[41] Jacobs B, Fornal C. Serotonin and behaviour, a general hypothesis. In: Bloom F, Kupfer DJ, editors. Psychopharmacology, the fourth generation in progress. New York: Raven Press; 1995. p. 461-9.

[42] Mortensen JT, Olsen J, Larsen H, Bendsen J, Obel C, Sorensen HT. Psychomotor development in children exposed in utero to benzodiazepines, antidepressants, neuroleptics, and anti-epileptics. *Eur. J. Epidemiol.* 2003;18(8):769-71.

[43] Misri S, Reebye P, Kendrick K, Carter D, Ryan D, Grunau RE, et al. Internalizing behaviors in 4-year-old children exposed in utero to psychotropic medications. *Am. J. Psychiatry* 2006 Jun;163(6):1026-32.

[44] Oberlander TF, Reebye P, Misri S, Papsdorf M, Kim J, Grunau RE. Externalizing and attentional behaviors in children of depressed mothers treated with a selective serotonin reuptake inhibitor antidepressant during pregnancy. *Arch. Pediatr. Adolesc. Med.* 2007 Jan;161(1):22-9.

[45] Oberlander TF, Papsdorf M, Brain UM, Misri S, Ross C, Grunau RE. Prenatal effects of selective serotonin reuptake inhibitor antidepressants, serotonin transporter promoter genotype (SLC6A4), and maternal mood on child behavior at 3 years of age. *Archives of Pediatrics and Adolescent Medicine* 2010;164(5):444.

[46] Reebye P, Morison SJ, Panikkar H, Misri S, Grunau R. Affect expression in prenatally psychotropic exposed and nonexposed mother-infant dyads. *Infant Mental Health Journal* 2002;23(4):403-16.

[47] Croen LA, Grether JK, Yoshida CK, Odouli R, Hendrick V. Antidepressant use during pregnancy and childhood autism spectrum disorders. *Arch. Gen. Psychiatry* 2011 Nov;68(11):1104-12.

[48] Kolevzon A, Gross R, Reichenberg A. Prenatal and perinatal risk factors for autism: a review and integration of findings. *Archives of Pediatrics and Adolescent Medicine* 2007;161(4):326.

[49] Gardener H, Spiegelman D, Buka SL. Perinatal and Neonatal Risk Factors for Autism: A Comprehensive Meta-analysis. *Pediatrics* 2011;128(2):344-55.

[50] Saper CB. Brain Stem Modulation of Sensation, Movement, and Conciousness. In: Kandel ER, Schwartz JH, Jessell TM, editors. Principles of Neural Science. Fourth ed. United States of America: McGraw-Hill; 2000. p. 889-908.

[51] Allman J. Evolving Brains. New York: Scientific American Library; 2000.

[52] Whitaker-Azmitia PM. Serotonin and Development*. *Handbook of Behavioral Neuroscience*; 21:309-23.

[53] Pawluski JL. Perinatal Selective Serotonin Reuptake Inhibitor Exposure: Impact on Brain Development and Neural Plasticity. *Neuroendocrinology* 2011.

[54] Allman JM. Evolving Brains. New York: Scientific American Library; 1999.

[55] Kandel ER, Schwartz JH, Jessell TM. Principles of neural science: McGraw-Hill New York; 2000.

[56] Cooper JR, Bloom FE, Roth RH. The Biochemical Basis of Neuropharmacology. Seventh ed. New York: Oxford University Press; 1996.

[57] Rice D, Barone Jr S. Critical periods of vulnerability for the developing nervous system: evidence from humans and animal models Environ Health Perspect 108 (suppl 3): 511â€"533. Find this article online 2000.

[58] Stanwood GD, Levitt P. The Effects of Monoamines on the Developing Nervous System. In: Nelson CA, Luciana M, editors. Handbook of Developmental Cognitive Neuroscience. Cambridge: MIT Press; 2008.

[59] Whitaker-Azmitia PM, Druse M, Walker P, Lauder JM. Serotonin as a developmental signal. *Behavioural brain research* 1996;73(1-2):19.

[60] Lauder JM. Ontogeny of the Serotonergic System in the Rat: Serotonin as a Developmental Signala. *Annals of the New York Academy of Sciences* 1990;600(1):297-313.

[61] Borue X, Chen J, Condron BG. Developmental effects of SSRIs: lessons learned from animal studies. *International Journal of Developmental Neuroscience*2007;25(6):341-7.

[62] Andrews MH, Matthews SG. Programming of the hypothalamo-pituitary-adrenal axis: serotonergic involvement. Stress: *The International Journal on the Biology of Stress*2004;7(1):15-27.

[63] Hendrick V, Stowe ZN, Altshuler LL, Hwang S, Lee E, Haynes D. Placental passage of antidepressant medications. *Am. J. Psychiatry*2003 May;160(5):993-6.

[64] Rampono J, Proud S, Hackett LP, Kristensen JH, Ilett KF. A pilot study of newer antidepressant concentrations in cord and maternal serum and possible effects in the neonate. *Int. J. Neuropsychopharmacol.* 2004 Sep;7(3):329-34.

[65] Oberlander TF, Warburton W, Misri S, Aghajanian J, Hertzman C. Effects of timing and duration of gestational exposure to serotonin reuptake inhibitor antidepressants: population-based study. *Br. J. Psychiatry.* 2008 May;192(5):338-43.

[66] Levinson-Castiel R, Merlob P, Linder N, Sirota L, Klinger G. Neonatal abstinence syndrome after in utero exposure to selective serotonin reuptake inhibitors in term infants. *Archives of Pediatrics and Adolescent Medicine* 2006;160(2):173.

[67] Mulder EJH, Ververs FFT, de Heus R, Visser GHA. Selective serotonin reuptake inhibitors affect neurobehavioral development in the human fetus. *Neuropsychopharmacology* 2011;36(10):1961-71.

[68] Mayes LC, Ward A. Principles of Neurobehavioural Teratology. In: Cicchetti D, Walker EF, editors. Neurodevelopmental Mechanisms in Psychopathology. Cambridge: Cambridge University Press; 2003. p. 3-34.

[69] Edwards JG. Unwanted effects of psychotropic drugs 2: Drug interactions, effects during pregnancy and breast feeding, pharmaco-vigilance and medico-legal considerations. In: King DJ, editor. Seminars

in Clincal Psychopharmacology. Second ed. London: *Royal College of Psychiatrists*; 2005. p. 601-61.

[70] Rayen I, van den Hove DL, Prickaerts J, Steinbusch HW, Pawluski JL. Fluoxetine during Development Reverses the Effects of Prenatal Stress on Depressive-Like Behavior and Hippocampal Neurogenesis in Adolescence. *PLoS One* 2011;6(9):e24003.

[71] Hodes GE, Hill-Smith TE, Suckow RF, Cooper TB, Lucki I. Sex-specific effects of chronic fluoxetine treatment on neuroplasticity and pharmacokinetics in mice. Journal *of Pharmacology and Experimental Therapeutics* 2010;332(1):266-73.

[72] Lee LJ. Neonatal fluoxetine exposure affects the neuronal structure in the somatosensory cortex and somatosensory-related behaviors in adolescent rats. *Neurotoxicity research* 2009;15(3):212-23.

[73] Swerts CAS, Costa AMDD, Esteves A, Borato CES, Swerts MSO. Effects of fluoxetine and imipramine in rat fetuses treated during a critical gestational period: a macro and microscopic study. *Revista Brasileira de Psiquiatria* 2010;32(2):152-8.

[74] Vorhees CV, Acuff-Smith KD, Schilling MA, Fisher JE, Moran MS, Buelke-Sam J. A developmental neurotoxicity evaluation of the effects of prenatal exposure to fluoxetine in rats. *Toxicological Sciences* 1994;23(2):194-205.

[75] Lee HJ, Kim JW, Yim SV, Kim MJ, Kim SA, Kim YJ, et al. Fluoxetine enhances cell proliferation and prevents apoptosis in dentate gyrus of maternally separated rats. *Mol. Psychiatry* 2001 Nov;6(6):610, 725-8.

[76] Pawluski JL, Galea LAM, Brain U, Papsdorf M, Oberlander TF. Neonatal S100B protein levels after prenatal exposure to selective serotonin reuptake inhibitors. *Pediatrics* 2009;124(4):e662-e70.

[77] Devlin AM, Brain U, Austin J, Oberlander TF. Prenatal exposure to maternal depressed mood and the MTHFR C677T variant affect SLC6A4 methylation in infants at birth. *PLoS One* 2010;5(8):e12201.

[78] Bairy K, Madhyastha S, Ashok K, Bairy I, Malini S. Developmental and behavioral consequences of prenatal fluoxetine. *Pharmacology-Basel-2007*;79(1):1.

[79] Zusso M, Debetto P, Guidolin D, Barbierato M, Manev H, Giusti P. Fluoxetine-induced proliferation and differentiation of neural progenitor cells isolated from rat postnatal cerebellum. *Biochemical pharmacology* 2008;76(3):391-403.

[80] Laine K, Heikkinen T, Ekblad U, Kero P. Effects of exposure to selective serotonin reuptake inhibitors during pregnancy on serotonergic

symptoms in newborns and cord blood monoamine and prolactin concentrations. *Arch. Gen. Psychiatry* 2003 Jul;60(7):720-6.

[81]   Oberlander TF, Bonaguro RJ, Misri S, Papsdorf M, Ross CJ, Simpson EM. Infant serotonin transporter (SLC6A4) promoter genotype is associated with adverse neonatal outcomes after prenatal exposure to serotonin reuptake inhibitor medications. *Mol. Psychiatry* 2008 Jan;13(1):65-73.

[82]   Anderson GM, Czarkowski K, Ravski N, Epperson CN. Platelet serotonin in newborns and infants: ontogeny, heritability, and effect of in utero exposure to selective serotonin reuptake inhibitors. *Pediatric research* 2004;56(3):418.

[83]   Epperson CN, Jatlow PI, Czarkowski K, Anderson GM. Maternal fluoxetine treatment in the postpartum period: effects on platelet serotonin and plasma drug levels in breastfeeding mother-infant pairs. *Pediatrics* 2003;112(5):e425.

[84]   Ansorge MS, Zhou M, Lira A, Hen R, Gingrich JA. Early-life blockade of the 5-HT transporter alters emotional behaviour in adult mice. *Science* 2004;306:879-81.

[85]   Lisboa S, Oliveira P, Costa L, Venâncio E, Moreira E. Behavioral evaluation of male and female mice pups exposed to fluoxetine during pregnancy and lactation. *Pharmacology* 2007;80(1):49.

[86]   Kusakawa S, Nakamura K, Miyamoto Y, Sanbe A, Torii T, Yamauchi J, et al. Fluoxetine promotes gliogenesis during neural differentiation in mouse embryonic stem cells. *Journal of neuroscience research* 2010;88(16):3479-87.

[87]   Maciag D, Simpson KL, Coppinger D, Lu Y, Wang Y, Lin RCS, et al. Neonatal antidepressant exposure has lasting effects on behavior and serotonin circuitry. *Neuropsychopharmacology* 2005;31(1):47-57.

[88]   Weaver KJ, Paul IA, Lin R, Simpson KL. Neonatal Exposure to Citalopram Selectively Alters the Expression of the Serotonin Transporter in the Hippocampus: Doseâ€• Dependent Effects. The Anatomical Record: *Advances in Integrative Anatomy and Evolutionary Biology*2010.

[89]   Olivier JDA, Vallès A, van Heesch F, Afrasiab-Middelman A, Roelofs JJPM, Jonkers M, et al. Fluoxetine administration to pregnant rats increases anxiety-related behavior in the offspring. *Psychopharmacology* 2011:1-14.

[90]   Vartazarmian R, Malik S, Baker GB, Boksa P. Long-term effects of fluoxetine or vehicle administration during pregnancy on behavioral

outcomes in guinea pig offspring. *Psychopharmacology* (Berl)2005 Mar;178(2-3):328-38.

[91] Gluckman PD, Hanson MA. The Developmental Origins of Health and Disease. *Early Life Origins of Health and Disease*2006:1-7.

[92] Goldberg AD, Allis CD, Bernstein E. Epigenetics: A landscape takes shape. *Cell* 2007;128(4):635-8.

[93] Van den Bergh BRH, Mulder EJH, Mennes M, Glover V. Antenatal maternal anxiety and stress and the neurobehavioural development of the fetus and child: links and possible mechanisms. A review. *Neuroscience and Biobehavioral Reviews* 2005;29(2):237-58.

[94] O'Donnell K, Bugge JA, Freeman L, Khalife N, O'Connor T, Glover V. Maternal prenatal anxiety and downregulation of placental 11Î²-HSD2. *Psychoneuroendocrinology* 2011.

[95] Glover V, O'Connor T, O'Donnell K. Prenatal stress and the programming of the HPA axis. *Neuroscience and Biobehavioral Reviews* 2010;35(1):17-22.

In: Antidepressants
Editors: L. J. Mígne and J. W. Post

ISBN: 978-1--62081-555-7
© 2012 Nova Science Publishers, Inc.

Chapter 2

ADDICTIVE POTENTIALS OF ANTIDEPRESSANT DRUGS

*R. Bou Khalil**

Psychiatric Hospital of the Cross- Jalledib- Lebanon,
Saint Joseph University, Beirut, Lebanon

ABSTRACT

Antidepressant drugs are relatively efficient psychopharmacologic agents that are widely used in the treatment of anxiety and affective disorders although controversies are attached to their adverse reactions' profile. In particular, the possibility of this family of drugs to withhold addictive potentials has not been profoundly studied in the literature although it might be encountered in daily clinical practice. In fact, many case reports described antidepressant drug abuse or dependence such as in the case of misuse of antidepressant drugs having amphetamine-like properties. Misuse of antidepressants concern mainly patients with a diagnosis of personality disorder and a previous history of drug or alcohol abuse and who are treated for a depressive disorder. Methadone treated patients are often prone to antidepressant drugs misuse. The latter may enhance the rewarding effect of other psychoactive drugs. From a neurobiological perspective, antidepressant drugs act on the same monoamines involved in addiction. Conversely, the pharmacodynamic

* Corresponding author: Rami BOU KHALIL, M.D. Psychiatric Hospital of the Cross- Jalledib- Lebanon, Saint Joseph University- Beirut- Lebanon. Tel: 0096170946430. E-mail: ramiboukhalil@hotmail.com.

profiles of most antidepressants and the absence of acute "desirable" effects in therapeutic dosages make addiction theoretically unlikely. However, rare cases of antidepressant drugs misuse exist in the literature. Discontinuation syndrome and tachyphylaxis/ tolerance are both frequently encountered aspects of antidepressant drugs usage. They correspond to the physical component of the dependence on this class of drugs and are in no means sufficient or indicative of a predisposition or a presence of a dependence on antidepressant drugs. Accordingly, their occurrence should never be confounded with the very rare typical dependence on antidepressant drugs. In this chapter, a review of the literature intends to cover all aspects of this controversial issue regarding antidepressant drugs safety.

1. INTRODUCTION

The search for substances altering the consciousness and improving mood is an important human trait. Addiction is a syndrome in which the hallmark is a compulsive pattern of drug use. Antidepressant drugs are relatively efficient psychopharmacologic agents that are widely used in the treatment of anxiety and affective disorders although controversies are attached to their adverse reactions' profile. Medical authorities do not regard antidepressants as causing addiction or dependence. However, far from being infrequent, the public views toward antidepressant drugs consider them to be addictive agents [1, 2]. In a survey from Denmark, 56% of respondents agreed that "your body can become addicted to antidepressants" and the same percentage thought that "when you have taken antidepressants over a long period of time it is difficult to stop taking them" [3]. As a matter of fact, the terms dependence and addiction carry a number of different meanings. Dependence itself has been divided into physical dependence used to cover the occurrence of tolerance and/or withdrawal symptoms and psychological dependence describing the range from craving to being reluctant to stop a drug for fear of becoming ill. According to DSM-IV-TR criteria, the diagnosis of dependence should be established when several aspects of dependence are present over a sufficient period of time (see table 1) [4]. In these criteria, physical signs and symptoms of dependence namely tolerance and withdrawal are not sufficient, alone, to establish the diagnosis of substance dependence. However, psychological signs and symptoms, when sufficient in number (three or more), are, by themselves, sufficient to confirm a diagnosis of substance dependence [4].

Table 1. Diagnostic criteria for substance dependence
as proposed by DSM-IV-TR [4]

Substance dependence: *A maladaptive pattern of substance use, leading to clinically significant impairment or distress, as manifested by three (or more) of the following, occurring at any time in the same 12-month period:*
(1) Tolerance, as defined by either of the following: (a) a need for markedly increased amounts of the substance to achieve Intoxication or desired effect (b) markedly diminished effect with continued use of the same amount of the substance (2) Withdrawal, as manifested by either of the following: (a) the characteristic withdrawal syndrome for the substance (refer to Criteria A and B of the criteria sets for withdrawal from the specific substances) (b) the same (or a closely related) substance is taken to relieve or avoid withdrawal symptoms (3) The substance is often taken in larger amounts or over a longer period than was intended (4) There is a persistent desire or unsuccessful efforts to cut down or control substance use (5) A great deal of time is spent in activities necessary to obtain the substance (e.g., visiting multiple doctors or driving long distances), use the substance (e.g., chain-smoking), or recover from its effects (6) Important social, occupational, or recreational activities are given up or reduced because of substance use (7) The substance use is continued despite knowledge of having a persistent or recurrent physical or psychological problem that is likely to have been caused or exacerbated by the substance.
Specify if: With Physiological Dependence: evidence of tolerance or withdrawal (i.e., either Item 1 or 2 is present) Without Physiological Dependence: no evidence of tolerance or withdrawal (i.e., neither Item 1 nor 2 is present)

A hierarchy of three key elements or "levels" to drug addiction has been proposed. It includes a level of physiological adaptation, a level of craving or abnormal desire for the drug and a level of failure of resolve called akrasia [5]. This approach shows that dependence and/or addiction involve a range of phenomena, from physiological effects through to cognitive and behavioral elements which renders drawing the line between the presence and the absence of a diagnosis of addiction and/or dependence quite difficult. However, the presence of either physical signs and/or symptoms of dependence such as tolerance and/or withdrawal, or of psychological signs and/or symptoms of dependence such as compulsiveness and drug seeking behavior should be sufficient to suspect the presence of addictive potentials for any psycho-active substance and particularly for antidepressant drugs. In this chapter, all aspects of the addictive potentials of antidepressant drugs will be reviewed in order to better address this problem when asked about or encountered in clinical settings.

2. ANTIDEPRESSANT DRUGS' DISCONTINUATION SYNDROME

Discontinuation symptoms are characteristic symptoms that follow termination or reduction in drug dosage, are self-limiting, reversed by re-introducing the drug and which cannot be explained as a reappearance of the disorder for which the drug was prescribed [6]. The pathogenesis of discontinuation syndrome remains controversial. It has been speculated that a temporary deficiency of synaptic serotonin with abrupt withdrawal of a serotoninergic antidepressant drug may explain the occurrence of a discontinuation syndrome after the drug discontinuation. This deficiency is compounded by the fact that down-regulated receptors will remain in their relatively hypoactive state for days to weeks. This is believed to result in antidepressant discontinuation syndrome directly or indirectly via downstream effects on other neurotransmitter systems (e.g., norepinephrine, dopamine, and γ-aminobutyric acid) implicated in depressive and anxiety disorders [7].

Discontinuation symptoms on withdrawal of tricyclic antidepressants are well described. They were first reported with imipramine [8-10]. Gastro-intestinal (abdominal pain, nausea, vomiting and diarrhea) and flu-like symptoms, fatigue, anxiety, psychomotor agitation, nightmares and sleep disturbances are the most common features. Movement disorders such as akathisia and behavioral activation with hypomania are occasional effects. Miscellaneous effects include cardiac arrhythmias. Most cases of switching to mania upon discontinuation of an antidepressant occur with tricyclic antidepressant drugs [11]. Controlled data on the prevalence of discontinuation symptoms are few, but long term therapy and abrupt withdrawal from a high daily dosage appear to be contributory factors. It has also been suggested that the antidepressants with stronger anticholinergic activity have more frequent and severe discontinuation symptoms associated with them but cholinergic agents have been found to be ineffective in relieving discontinuation symptoms [12]. Discontinuation symptoms have been described in 50% of patients suddenly stopping high-dose of imipramine, and in 30% of patients undergoing supervised withdrawal of clomipramine [13, 14].

Discontinuation syndromes with Mono-Amine Oxidase Inhibitors (MAOIs), particularly tranylcypromine, are usually more severe than with other antidepressants. Because MAOIs cause changes in the $\alpha2$-adrenergic and dopaminergic receptors, their discontinuation may cause agitation and psychosis. An acute confusional state with disorientation, paranoid delusions and hallucinations may occur [15]. A worsening of depressive symptoms, exceeding the severity of the state that originally led to treatment, is also recognized as is hypomania [16, 17]. Generalized seizures have been described following stoppage of tranylcypromine [18].

The initial selective serotonin reuptake inhibitor (SSRI) discontinuation syndrome was described for fluoxetine in 1988 [19]. Subsequent case reports and large studies documented its occurrence with all other SSRIs, primarily paroxetine [20-22]. A meta-analysis of all case reports and research published up to 1997 found that 30 of 46 cases (65%) were linked to paroxetine, compared with 8 (17%) for sertraline, 5 (11%) for fluoxetine, and 3 (7%) for fluvoxamine. The prevalence of the syndrome ranged from 7.2% with SSRIs with a short half-life (paroxetine and fluvoxamine) to as low as 2.2% with SSRIs with a longer half-life (sertraline and fluoxetine) [23]. One observational study found that four of 45 patients (9 %) given fluoxetine and 26 of 52 patients (50 %) given paroxetine reported discontinuation symptoms, with a mean onset of two days and mean duration of five days [24]. A randomized controlled trial (RCT) comparing three SSRIs found a lower incidence of antidepressant discontinuation syndrome with fluoxetine (14%) than with paroxetine (66%) or sertraline (60 %) [25]. In addition, a retrospective chart review of 350 patients using SSRIs showed no significant added risk associated with age, sex, or diagnosis [13]. Perhaps the best evidence comes from an RCT that found mild to moderate antidepressant discontinuation symptoms in 35% of patients given paroxetine and 14% given placebo who were abruptly withdrawn from treatment after 12 weeks. The difference of approximately 20 percent between active treatment and placebo for one of the drugs most commonly associated with antidepressant discontinuation syndrome may provide an upper boundary for the probability of the condition [26]. Clinical manifestations of SSRI discontinuation syndrome resemble those of TCA discontinuation syndrome with three additional symptom clusters (problems with balance, sensory abnormalities, aggressive and impulsive behavior) and without cardiac arrhythmias (see table 2) [27]. In the vast majority of patients, SSRI discontinuation symptoms occur within 1 to 3 days after cessation of treatment or reduction in dose [28]. In most cases, the discontinuation syndrome is mild and short-lived, even if untreated [13, 29]. Discontinuation symptoms are generally suppressed by re-introduction of the antidepressant, with subsequent tapering preventing their re-emergence. Accordingly, tapering over a period of at least four weeks, as opposed to abrupt stoppage, has been recommended as part of routine practice by several authorities [30-34].

Table 2. Diagnostic criteria for SSRI discontinuation syndrome as proposed by Black et al. 2000 [26]

Proposed diagnostic criteria for SSRI discontinuation syndrome:	
Criterion A	Discontinuation of or reduction in dose of an SSRI after a period of use of at least 1 month.
Criterion B	Two or more of the following symptoms developing after one to seven days of criterion A: Anxiety Diarrhea Fatigue Gait instability Headache Insomnia Irritability Nausea and/or emesis Tremor Visual disturbances
Criterion C	The symptoms in criterion B cause clinically significant distress or impairment in social, occupational or important areas of functioning
Criterion D	The symptoms are not due to a general medical condition and are not better accounted for by recurrence of symptoms of the mental disorder for which the SSRI was originally prescribed, or by concurrent discontinuation (or reduction in use) of another psycho-active substance

Discontinuation syndromes from other antidepressant drugs such as venlafaxine, duloxetine, mirtazapine and nefazodone have been also described [35-46]. Most frequent and relatively severe discontinuation syndrome seems to be related to venlafaxine which manifests clinically with headache, dizziness, nausea, diarrhea, akathisia, shock-like sensations and irregularities in blood pressure [35-41]. The incidence of venlafaxine discontinuation symptoms is considered to be 78% after the stoppage of the extended release formulation administered for a 6 to 10 week treatment period and a two week tapering period (as compared to 22% in placebo treated individuals) [36]. As for duloxetine, a pooled analysis of 6 short-term treatment trials, in which treatment was stopped abruptly, discontinuation emergent adverse events were reported by 44.3% of duloxetine- treated patients (as compared to 22.9% of placebo-treated patients) [43].

In conclusion, discontinuation syndrome is a frequent clinical entity occurring after the discontinuation of nearly every concurrently available antidepressant drug. However, it has been more frequently reported with the discontinuation of some antidepressant drugs with a short half-life such as paroxetine and venlafaxine. It has also been more frequently reported when antidepressant drug has been stopped abruptly after being taken for a long period. The presence of a discontinuation syndrome after antidepressant drug stoppage does not implicate that the patient has developed a dependence on the antidepressant drug stopped, unless this discontinuation syndrome has been accompanied with symptoms of tolerance (or tachyphylaxis as it will be exposed in the next section) and/or of psychological dependence with drug seeking behavior.

3. TOLERANCE OR TACHYPHYLAXIS TOWARD ANTIDEPRESSANT DRUGS

The pharmacological term *tachyphylaxis,* introduced by Leib and Balter in 1984, is defined as a rapid appearance of progressive decrease in response to a given dose after repetitive administration of a pharmacologically or physiologically active substance [47, 48]. In many studies antidepressant drugs tachyphylaxis (or "poop-out" effect) is defined as a relapse or recurrence of an episode of major depression after full recovery from a major depressive episode despite continued treatment with a previously effective antidepressant [49]. It has been suggested that a more appropriate term for this phenomenon should be antidepressant tolerance [50]. Antidepressant drugs tachyphylaxis/ tolerance is characterized by symptoms of apathy or decreased motivation, fatigue, dullness in cognitive function, sleep disturbance, weight gain, and sexual dysfunction with patients stating that they feel worse than they felt after initially achieving remission on the antidepressant, but not as bad as they felt before treatment initiation [52]. Moreover, this phenomenon is distinguished from relapse or recurrence by the fact that the former always occurs under continuous antidepressant drug intake.

The incidence of antidepressant tachyphylaxis/ tolerance is still unknown but has been estimated according to published trials to range between 9% and 33% which correspond to the frequency of return of depressive symptoms during maintenance antidepressant treatment in full dosage [52]. In a double-blind crossover study, 31% of depressed patients who responded to placebo showed symptoms of possible tachyphylaxis in the 7- to 12-week follow-up period while only 12% of imipramine-responders and approximately 9% who were taking phenelzine were suspected of developing tolerance [53]. In a prospective study, tachyphylaxis occurred in 25% of treatments followed over a period of mean duration of 20 weeks, with a two-fold risk elevation in cases of melancholic depression [49]. In a retrospective study, rates of tachyphylaxis were significantly lower with venlafaxine and tricyclic antidepressant drugs (3.7%) compared to rates of tachyphylaxis with SSRIs (14.1%) [54]. In another prospective study in which SSRI were excluded, only 3.8% of tachyphylxis were reported in 59 patients suffering from a major depressive disorder with psychotic features followed over a 4 month period [55]. In a review of medical case reports, tachyphylaxis/ tolerance cases were most frequently found in female subjects having a mean age of 42 years old [52].

Causes of tachyphylaxis/tolerance are not well understood but some explanations are available. Of those, non-adherence and loss of placebo effect have been considered as factors unrelated to effects on neurons [56]. Several genetic polymorphisms have been associated with therapeutic SSRI response and may accordingly be incriminated in lack of response to this class of drugs [57-59]. In addition, serotonin receptor desensitization has been hypothesized to be the primary actor responsible for the observation of an increased risk for the return of depressive symptoms during long-term treatment with SSRI as well as with repeated antidepressant drug administration [60, 61]. Some studies showed that tachyphylaxis/tolerance is more common in patients suffering from bipolar type II major depressive disorder so that cases of rapid response to antidepressant drugs followed by a poop-out period may correspond to an initial phase of mood switch [62]. Other explanations such as tolerance related to pharmacokinetic fluctuations in antidepressant drugs effect, their possible prophylactic inefficacy as well as their possible attributed paradoxical effect have also been proposed [52, 59, 63].

Management of tachyphylaxis/ tolerance to antidepressant drug has not been well studied in the literature. In addition, the definitions of tachyphylaxis/ tolerance and relapse may have been considered interchangeable in the studies that have been interested to the subject. In face of a tachyphylaxis/ tolerance to an antidepressant drug, it may be intuitive to augment its dosage in order to reinstall the initial response to the medication. In a survey where 145 psychiatrists specialized in psychopharmacology of affective disorders participated, the most popular choice in front of a hypothetical breakthrough depression in patients under antidepressant drugs was increasing the dosage [64]. As a part of a placebo-controlled study, 18 patients who suffered from possible tachyphylaxis on fluoxetine 20 mg/day during long-term treatment had their fluoxetine dose augmented to 40 mg/day and were followed for at least 1 month. Among those patients 67% were full responders, 17% partial responders and 17% dropped out because of side effects. 61% of patients maintained their response during their follow-up period (mean duration = 4.7 months). It has been concluded that an increase in dose of fluoxetine to 40 mg/day appears to be an effective strategy in the treatment of the tachy-phylaxis/ tolerance of fluoxetine in dosage of 20 mg/day [65]. However, in 4 cases lowering the dosage of fluoxetine after a washout period seemed to improve the response to this antidepressant drug [66].

In conclusion, tachyphylaxis/ tolerance to antidepressant drug effect is a frequently encountered aspect of this class of drugs usage. It seems to be more frequent with SSRIs than with other classes of antidepressant drugs. The presence of tachyphylaxis/ tolerance to a certain antidepressant drug does not implicate that the patient has developed a dependence on this particular drug. While it is true that the presence of tachyphylaxis/ tolerance might implicate that the antidepressant drug' dosage must be augmented this is not indicative of a predisposition to develop dependence unless it was accompanied with other symptoms such as a discontinuation syndrome and/or symptoms of psychological dependence. Whenever dosage augmentation is considered it is generally circumscribed under medical monitoring. It cannot be considered as an indicator of dependence unless the patient develops a self-medication behavior and/or inadequately seeks medically assisted antidepressant dosage augmentation. Moreover, due to the relatively high incidence of both discontinuation syndrome and tachyphylaxis/tolerance, one can expect that their coexistence in a particular patient is a frequent encounter. This corresponds to the patient who initially responds to a certain antidepressant drug but develops tachyphylaxis/ tolerance after several weeks and continues afterwards to become tolerant to every subsequent escalating dosage of the antidepressant drug. When the administered antidepressant drug is tapered down, discontinuation symptoms preclude its total stoppage in a way that a combination of antidepressant drugs remains the only solution. Although publically considered as a form of dependence, similar situations are far from being considered as such unless discontinuation syndrome remains resistant to every tapering strategy and psychological dependence signs and symptoms exist.

4. PSYCHOLOGICAL DEPENDENCE ON ANTIDEPRESSANT DRUGS

Psychological signs and symptoms of dependence on a psycho-active substance have been defined in the DSM-IV-TR in the following simplified way (for further details see table 1) [4]:

a. Substance used differently than intended
b. Loss of control on substance usage while desiring to regain it
c. Excessive time spent obtaining, using or recovering
    from effects of substance
d. Substance use takes priority over daily life functioning
e. Substance use continues despite persistent or recurrent harm

As previously mentioned, the presence of psychological dependence (as related to the presence of three of the above symptoms during a period of at least twelve months) is sufficient to confirm the diagnosis of dependence on a certain substance. In the particular case of antidepressant drugs, no specific clinical study evaluating the presence of equivalent psychological signs and symptoms of dependence in patients receiving antidepressant drugs exist. However, the prevalence of drug dependence on SSRI has been evaluated to be 0.1% according to the data base of the United Kingdom adverse drug reaction reports examined by the medicines control agency [67].

A broader concept of substance misuse has been defined in the DSM-IV-TR criteria (see table 3) [4]. Substance abuse is only diagnosed if the patient does not fulfill further criteria for the diagnosis of substance dependence.

**Table 3. Definition criteria for substance abuse according
to the DSM-IV-TR classification [4]**

Substance Abuse:
A maladaptive pattern of substance use leading to clinically significant impairment or distress, as manifested by one (or more) of the following, occurring within a 12-month period:
Recurrent substance use resulting in a failure to fulfill major role obligations at work, school, or home (e.g., repeated absences or poor work performance related to substance use; substance-related absences, suspensions or expulsions from school; neglect of children or household) Recurrent substance use in situations in which it is physically hazardous (e.g., driving an automobile or operating a machine when impaired by substance use) Recurrent substance-related legal problems (e.g., arrests for substance-related disorderly conduct) Continued substance use despite having persistent or recurrent social or interpersonal problems caused or exacerbated by the effects of the substance (e.g., arguments with spouse about consequences of intoxication, physical fights)
The symptoms have never met the criteria for Substance Dependence for this class of substance.

One study has evaluated the prevalence of antidepressant drug abuse in 225 patients hospitalized for treatment of prescription drug abuse. Of 453 abused prescription drugs, 10 were antidepressant drugs. In no case was the antidepressant drug the main drug of abuse [68].

Data related to the antidepressant drugs class' potential of being misused emanate essentially from case reports and series. Case reports of patients abusing or becoming dependant on antidepressant drugs are numerous in the literature. Accordingly, psychological dependence on this class of drugs may be better understood via a thorough evaluation of these reports. In a review of those of them published before 1998, 35 case reports of antidepressant drug misuse (dependence or abuse) were identified among which 21 case reports of dependence existed. These reports were restricted to five agents, and dominated by the central nervous system stimulating drug tranylcypromine (12/21) and the dopaminergic tricyclic antidepressant drug amineptine (4/21) which is unlicensed in many countries. The remaining five reports were for nomifensine, fluoxetine or amitriptyline. Most cases corresponded to male patients (14/21), who had a history of prior substance abuse (14/21) or personality disorders (10/21). Tolerance often occurred leading to exceptionally high dosages, sometimes more than 10-fold higher than that prescribed. Several patients consulted multiple doctors to ensure supplies. The commonest reason given for misuse was to obtain a stimulant effect and most such patients (6/8) had a prior history of stimulant misuse. Other reasons given for misuse were to improve work/social functioning (n=5) and to lift mood/keep well (n=4) and to obtain a euphoriant effect (n=4) [67].

In the modern literature, a few case reports of dependence on antidepressant drugs exist while many case reports of antidepressant drug abuse exist. In a case report, a 45 year old man with no personal psychiatric history has been considered to have a dependence on amineptine which effect was lessened with midazolam. He has been put on antidepressant drug after going through stressful life events. Amineptine gave him a sense of "decisiveness" and increased speed of thinking. From experimentation, he discovered the pleasurable effect of amineptine. His daily intake increased from 200 mg/day to 2000 mg/day within a few weeks. Of note, the diagnosis of amineptine dependence has not been made according to DSM-IV-TR criteria [69]. Another case described a 34 year old woman with no psychiatric history other than a post-traumatic stress disorder for which she had received 37.5 mg/day of the tricyclic antidepressant tianeptine. She reinitiated this treatment by herself a few years later when she was going through stressful life events but reached 750 mg/day because of discontinuation and tolerance symptoms. She was also seeking a feeling of being "better and strong" after tianeptine intake [70]. A third case report described a 53 year old man with a psychiatric history of borderline personality disorder, alcohol dependence and amineptine abuse. He augmented, by himself, the prescribed dose of 75 mg/day of venlafaxine for a major depressive episode to a maximum of 50 tablets per day (3750 mg/day). During his high levels of venlafaxine intake, he reported feeling more empathic and sociable and having an elated mood [71]. Other case reports of antidepressant drugs misuse from more recent literature concern cases of antidepressant drug abuse. Those reports concern older antidepressant drugs, such as tianeptine, as well as newer antidepressant drugs, such as the dopaminergic agent bupropion. Some atypical features of those antidepressant drugs abuse, such as nasal insufflations are becoming more and more recognized [72-75].

In conclusion, psychological signs and symptoms of dependence on an antidepressant drug are a prerequisite for the establishment of such a diagnosis. Patients suffering from one or more symptoms because of which their excessive consumption of antidepressant drug may impair their social, professional and relational functioning and/or endanger their or other's physical health are considered to have antidepressant drug abuse. When these symptoms exist with other psychological symptoms such as loss of control over antidepressant usage and/or physical symptoms such tachyphylaxis/ tolerance and discontinuation, patients are considered to have antidepressant drug dependence. Typical cases of antidepressant drug dependence concern patients with a comorbid personality disorder and a history of other substance misuse. Stimulant antidepressant drugs are most frequently misused for their mood elating and self-confidence reinforcing effects. The differentiation between dependence and abuse of psycho-active substances seems to have lowered the frequency of case reports of patients suffering from antidepressant drug dependence in favor of those suffering from antidepressant drug abuse. As a matter of fact, drug seeking behavior and compulsiveness of intake (which may be presented in the third, fourth and fifth criteria of the DSM-IV-TR diagnostic criteria of substance dependence) are not easily applicable when the concerned psycho-active drug is an antidepressant. These drugs are most frequently prescribed under medical monitoring and do not exert any researched effect unless they were taken in very high doses. Accordingly, it may seem more feasible, for a patient who is seeking some psychological benefit from antidepressant drug misuse, to abuse them rather than becoming dependant on them. However, due to their previously described properties such as discontinuation syndrome and tachyphylaxis/ tolerance a very small proportion of patients who are originally prone to misuse them, may develop a typical dependence on them.

5. NEUROBIOLOGICAL RATIONALE BEHIND ANTIDEPRESSANT DRUG DEPENDENCE

Psycho-active substance addiction may be regarded as the disease of the brain reward system. This system, closely related to the system of emotional arousal, is located predominantly in the limbic structures of the brain. All addictive drugs have in common that they enhance dopaminergic reward synaptic function in the nucleus accumbens. The anatomical core of the reward system are dopaminergic neurons of the ventral tegmentum that project, via the medial forebrain bundle, to the nucleus accumbens, amygdala, ventral pallidum, prefrontal cortex and other forebrain structures. Addiction appears to correlate with a hypodopaminergic dysfunctional state within the reward circuitry of the brain. It progresses from occasional recreational use to impulsive use to habitual compulsive use and is related to the occurrence of the "desirable" psychological effects after single doses [76, 77].

In human and animal models, it has been demonstrated that most antidepressants have no such effect although imipramine, for example, has been shown to induce a transient euphoric state [78-80]. Data concerning antidepressant drug abuse in combination with methadone exist. This misuse potential of antidepressant drugs in patients receiving methadone as a maintenance treatment is the result of pharmacodynamic interactions between both compounds. For example, desipramine plasma levels are increased by methadone. Furthermore, fluvoxamine and fluoxetine to a lesser extent may cause an important increase in serum methadone concentrations. The inhibition of different clusters of the cytochrome P450 system is also involved in these interactions [81]. On another hand, antidepressant drugs in combination with methadone as well as other opioids have been shown to enhance pain relief [82, 83]. More specifically, serotonin uptake inhibitors have been shown to selectively enhance the antinociceptive effects of opioid receptor agonists in nonhuman primates when combined to these agonists but not when used alone [83]. Early studies have demonstrated that patients receiving methadone maintenance treatment find the combination of methadone from one side and amitriptyline or dothiepin from another side enabling them to achieve euphoria [84, 85]. More recently, high prevalences of amitriptyline abuse were found in patients receiving methadone maintenance treatment and needle-exchanging subjects (26% and 15.8% respectively) [86, 87].

Pharmacodynamic properties needed for any psycho-active substance in order for it to be considered as potentially addictive, are not met in the case of most antidepressant drugs although some exceptions may exist. Dopamine enhancing antidepressant drugs may resemble in their mechanism of action cocaine and amphetamines. This amphetamine-like effect is minor unless these antidepressant drugs were taken in enormous quantities. Antidepressant drugs having amphetamine-like effects are atypical tricyclic drugs having an action of dopamine such amineptine, tianeptine, MAOIs such as tranylcypromine, and among newer antidepressant drugs the dopamine reuptake inhibitor bupropion [88-91].

In conclusion, a neurobiological rationale supporting the addictive potential of antidepressant drugs exists although it requires the presence of one of two conditions: First, the antidepressant drug, especially tricylic antidepressant drugs, has to be abused in combination with opioid agonists.

Second, the antidepressant drug, especially those with amphetamine-like properties, has to be consumed in high dosages.

CONCLUSION

A categorical refute of the presence of addictive potentials when talking about antidepressant drugs seems to be a hasty approach to this aspect of these drugs' adverse effects. A careful differentiation between, from one part, symptoms of discontinuation and tachyphylaxis/ tolerance and, from another part, symptoms of misuse, is crucial for a better management of both types of symptoms in a clinical setting. Patients may frequently be reluctant to receive antidepressant drugs, or even be poorly compliant to these medications, because of what is publically known about their potential addictive effect. Addictive potentials have to be clearly separated between antidepressant drugs potentials to be abused and their potential to cause dependence. Patients may be predisposed to become typically dependent on antidepressant drugs in extremely rare situations. In these situations, dependent individuals consume massive amounts of antidepressant drugs daily in a research for a certain mood elating effect while expressing other psychological symptoms such as compulsiveness in accompaniment with possible physical dependence symptoms such as tachyphylaxis/ tolerance and or discontinuation syndrome. Antidepressant drugs abuse, although a relatively rare complication seems to be more frequent than typical antidepressant drug dependence. In general, misused antidepressant drugs have amphetamine-like effect and/or are used in combination with opioid agonists. Patients predisposed to develop antidepressant drug misuse have most frequently a history of other psychoactive drugs misuse and/ or a personality disorder. Discontinuation syndrome and tachyphylaxis/ tolerance are both frequently encountered aspects of antidepressant drugs usage. They correspond to the physical component of the dependence on this class of drugs and are in no means sufficient or indicative of a predisposition or a presence of a dependence on antidepressant drugs. Accordingly, their occurrence should never be confounded with the very rare typical dependence on antidepressant drugs unless the patient develops, concomitantly, psychological symptoms of dependence.

REFERENCES

[1]   Priest, RG, Vize C, Roberts, A, Roberts, M, Tylee, A. Lay people's attitudes to treatment of depression: results of opinion poll for Defeat Depression Campaign just before its launch. *BMJ*, 1996, 313: 858-859.

[2]   Gray R, Plummer S, Ritter S Sandford T, Ritter S, Mundt-Leach R, Goldberg D, Gournay K. National survey of practice nurses. *J. Advanced Nursing*, 1999, 30: 901-906.

[3]   Kessing LV, Hansen HV, Demyttenaere K, Bech P. Depressive and bipolar disorders: patients' attitudes and beliefs towards depression and antidepressants. *Psychological Medicine*, 2005, 35: 1205-1213.

[4]   American Psychiatric Association. Diagnostic and statistical manual of mental disorders text revision (DSM-IV-TR). Fourth edition. Washington, DC: *American Psychiatric Association*; 2000.

[5]   Heather, N. A conceptual framework for explaining drug addiction. *Journal of psychopharmacology*, 1998, 12: 3-7.

[6]   Schatzberg AF, Haddad P, Kaplan EM, Lejoyeux, M, Rosenbaum, JF, Young, AH, Zajecka, J. Serotonin reuptake inhibitor discontinuation syndrome: a hypothetical definition. *Journal of clinical psychiatry*, 1997, 58: 5-10.

[7]   Lane, RM. Withdrawal symptoms after discontinuation of selective serotonin reuptake inhibitors (SSRIs). *Journal of serotonin research*, 1996, 3/2:75-83.

[8]   Manna, M, Macpherson, AS. Clinical experience with imipramine in the treatment of depression. *Canadian psychiatric association Journal*, 1959, 4: 3847.

[9]   Andersen, H, Kristiansen, ES. Tofranil treatment of endogenous depressions. *Acta psychiatrica scandinavica* 1959, 34: 386-397.

[10] Kramer, JC , Klein, DF, Fink, M . Withdrawal symptoms following discontinuation of imipramine therapy. *American Journal of psychiatry*, 1961, 118: 549-550.

[11] Ali, S, Milev, R. Switch to mania upon discontinuation of antidepressants in patients with mood disorders: a review of the literature. *Canadian Journal of Psychiatry*, 2003, 48: 258-264.

[12] Disalver, SC. Withdrawal phenomena associated with antidepressant and antipsychotic agents. *Drug safety*, 1994, 10: 103-114.

[13] Coupland, NJ, Bell, CJ, Potokar, JP. Serotonin reuptake inhibitor withdrawal. *Journal of clinical psychopharmacology*, 1996, 16: 356-362.

[14] Dilsaver, SC, Greden, JF . Antidepressant withdrawal phenomena. *Biological psychiatry*, 1984, 19: 237-256.

[15] Liskin, B, Roose, S, Walsh, T. Acute psychosis following phenelzine discontinuation. *Journal of clinical psychopharmacology*, 1984, 5: 46-47. .

[16] Halle, MT, Dilsaver, SC. Tranylcypromine withdrawal phenomena. *Journal of psychiatry and neuroscience*, 1993, 18: 49-50.

[17] Rothschild, AJ. Mania after withdrawal of isocarboxazid. *Journal of clinical psychopharmacology*, 1985, 5: 340-342.

[18] Vartzopulos, D, Krull, F. Dependence on monoamine oxidase inhibitors in high dose. *Bristish journal of psychiatry*, 1991, 158: 856-857.

[19] Cooper, GL. The safety of fluoxetine: an update. *British Journal of psychiatry,*1988, 153: 77-86.

[20] Black, K, Shea, C, Dursun, S, Kutcher, S. Selective serotonin reuptake inhibitor discontinuation syndrome: proposed diagnostic criteria. *Journal of psychiatry and neuroscience*, 2000, 25:255-261.

[21] Hindmarch, I, Kimber, S, Cockle, SM. Abrupt and brief discontinuation of antidepressant treatment: effects on cognitive function and psychomotor performance. *International clinical psychopharmacology*, 2000, 15: 305-318.

[22] Michelson, D, Fava, M, Amsterdam, J, Apter, J, Londborg, P, Tamura, R, Tepner, RG. Interruption of selective serotonin reuptake inhibitor treatment. *British Journal of psychiatry*, 2000, 176: 363-368.

[23] Black, K, Shea, C, Dursun, S, Kutcher, S. Selective serotonin reuptake inhibitor discontinuation syndrome: proposed diagnostic criteria. *Journal of psychiatry and neuroscience*, 2000, 25: 255-261.

[24] Bogetto, F, Bellino, S, Revello, RB, Patria, L. Discontinuation syndrome in dysthymic patients treated with selective serotonin reuptake inhibitors: a clinical investigation. *CNS drugs*, 2002, 16: 273-283.

[25] Rosenbaum, JF, Fava, M, Hoog, SL, Ascroft, RC, Krebs, WB. Selective serotonin reuptake inhibitor discontinuation syndrome: a randomized clinical trial. *Biological psychiatry*, 1998, 44: 77-87.

[26] Oehrberg, S, Christiansen, PE, Behnke, K, Borup, AL, Severin, B, Soegaard, J, Calberg, H, Judge, R, Ohrstrom, JK, Manniche, PM. Paroxetine in the treatment of panic disorder. A randomised, double-blind, placebo-controlled study. *British Journal of psychiatry*, 1995, 167: 374-379.

[27] Black, K, Shea, C, Dursun, S, Kutcher, S. Selective serotonin reuptake inhibitor discontinuation syndrome: proposed diagnostic criteria. *Journal of psychiatry and neuroscience*, 2000, 25: 255-261.

[28] Olver, JS, Burrows, GD, Norman, TR. Discontinuation syndromes with selective serotonin reuptake inhibitors. Are there clinically relevant differences? *CNS drugs*, 1999, 12: 171-177.

[29] Lejoyeux, M, Ades, J. Antidepressant discontinuation: a review of the literature. *Journal of clinical psychiatry*, 1997, 58: 11-16.

[30] Dominguez, RA, Goodnick, W. Adverse events after the abrupt discontinuation of paroxetine. *Pharmacotherapy*, 1995, 15: 778-780.

[31] Benazzi, F. Venlafaxine withdrawal symptoms. *Canadian Journal of psychiatry*, 1996, 41: 487-484.

[32] British Medical Association and Royal Pharmaceutical Society of Great Britain. *British National Formulary*, Section 4.3: Antidepressant drugs: withdrawal. London: The Pharmaceutical Press; 2000.

[33] Drug and Therapeutics Bulletin. Withdrawing patients from antidepressants. *Drug and therapeutics bulletin*, 1999, 37: 49-52.

[34] Rosenbaum, JF, Zajecka, J. Clinical management of antidepressant discontinuation. *Journal of clinical psychiatry*, 1997, 58: 37-40.

[35] Louie, AK, Lannon, RA, Kirsch, MA, Louis, TB. Venlafaxine withdrawal reactions. *American Journal of psychiatry*, 1996, 153: 1652.

[36] Fava, M, Mulroy, R, Alpert, J, Nierenberg, AA, Rosenbaum, JF. Emergence of adverse effects following discontinuation of treatment with extended-release venlafaxine. *American journal of psychiatry*, 1997, 154: 1760-1762.

[37] Giakas, WJ, Davis, SM. Intractable withdrawal from venlafaxine treated with fluoxetine. *Psychiatric annals*, 1997, 27: 85-86.

[38] Haddad, P. Newer antidepressant and the discontinuation syndrome. *Journal of clinical psychiatry*, 1997, 58: 17-22.

[39] Boyd, IW. Venlafaxine withdrawal reactions. *The med Journal of Australia*, 1998, 169:91-92.

[40] Sabljić, V, Ružić, K, Rakun, R. Venlafaxine withdrawal syndrome. *Psychiatria Danubina*, 2011, 23: 117-119.

[41] Koga, M, Kodaka, F, Miyata, H, Nakayama, K. Symptoms of delusion: the effects of discontinuation of low-dose venlafaxine. *Acta psychiatrica scandinavica*, 2009, 120: 329-331.

[42] Benazzi, F. Nefazodone withdrawal symptoms. *Candian journal of psychiatry*, 1998, 43: 194-195.

[43] Lauber, C. Nefazodone withdrawal symptoms. *Canadian Journal of psychiatry*, 1999, 44: 285-286.

[44] MacCall, C, Callender, J. Mirtazapine withdrawal causing hypomania. *British Journal psychiatry*, 1999, 175: 390.

[45] Perahia, DG, Kajdasz, DK, Desaiah, D, Haddad, PM. Symptoms following abrupt discontinuation of duloxetine treatment in patients with major depressive disorder. *Journal of affect disorders*, 2005, 89: 207-212.

[46] Pitchot, W, Ansseau, M. Shock-like sensations associated with duloxetine discontinuation. *Annals of clinical psychiatry*, 2008, 20: 175.

[47] Leib, J, Balter, A. Antidepressant tachyphylaxis. *Medical hypothesis*, 1984, 15: 279-291.

[48] Stedman, TL. *Stedman's Medical Dictionary*. 27th edition. Philadelphia: Lippincott, Williams, and Wilkins; 2000.

[49] Solomon, DA, Leon, AC, Mueller, TI, Coryell, W, Teres, JJ, Posternak, MA, Judd, LL, Endicott, J, Keller, MB. Tachyphylaxis in unipolar major depressive disorder. *Journal of clin psychiatry*, 2005, 66: 283-290.

[50] Byrne, S, Rothschild, A. Loss of antidepressant efficacy during maintenance therapy: Possible mechanisms and treatments. *Journal of clinical psychiatry*, 1998; 59: 279-288.

[51] Rothschild, A. The Rothschild Scale for Antidepressant Tachyphylaxis: Reliability and validity. *Comprehensive psychiatry*, 2008, 49: 508-513.

[52] Byrne, S, Rothschild, A. Loss of antidepressant efficacy during maintenance therapy: Possible mechanisms and treatments. *Journal of clinical psychiatry*, 1998, 59: 279-288.

[53] Quitkin, FM, Stewart, JW, McGrath, PJ, Nunes, E, Ocepek-Welikson, K, Tricamo, E, Rabkin, JG, Klein, DF. Further evidence that a placebo response to antidepressants can be identified. *American journal of psychiatry*, 1993, 150: 562-565.

[54] Posternak, MA, Zimmerman, M. Dual reuptake inhibitors incur lower rates of tachyphylaxis than selective serotonin reuptake inhibitors: A retrospective study. *Journal of clinical psychiatry*, 2005, 66: 705-707.

[55] Wijkstra, J, Burger, H, van den Broek, WW, Birkenhäger, TK, Janzing, JG, Boks, MP, Bruijn, JA, van der Loos, ML, Breteler, LM, Verkes, RJ, Nolen, WA. Long-term response to successful acute pharmacological treatment of psychotic depression. *Journal of affective disorders*, 2010, 123: 238-242.

[56] Kornstein, SG. Beyond remission, rationale, and design of the prevention of recurrent episodes of depression with venlafaxine for two years (PREVENT) Study. *CNS spectrums*, 2006, 11: 28-34.

[57] Neumeister, A, Hu, XZ, Luckenbaugh, DA, Schwarz, M, Nugent, AC, Bonne, O, Herscovitch, P, Goldman, D, Drevets, WC, Charney, DS. Differential effects of 5-HTTLPR genotypes on the behavioral and neural responses to tryptophan depletion in patients with major depression and controls. *Archives of general psychiatry*, 2006, 63: 978-986.

[58] Yoshimura, R, Hori, H, Ikenouchi-Sugita, A, Umene-Nakano, W, Ueda, N, Nakamura, J. Higher plasma interleukin-6 (IL-6) level is associated with SSRI- or SNRI-refractory depression. *Progress in neuropsychopharmacology and biological psychiatry*, 2009, 33: 722-726.

[59] Fava, GA. Can long-term treatment with antidepressant drugs worsen the course of depression? *Journal of clinical psychiatry*, 2003, 64: 123-133.

[60] Muraki, I, Inoue, T, Hashimoto, S, Izumi, T, Koyama, T. Effect of different challenge doses after repeated citalopram treatment on extracellular serotonin level in the medial prefrontal cortex: In vivo microdialysis study. *Psychiatry and clinical neuroscience*, 2008, 62: 568-574.

[61] Amsterdam, J, Williams, D, Michelson, D, Adler, LA, Dunner, DL, Nierenberg, AA, Reimherr, FW, Schatzberg, AF. Tachyphylaxis after repeated antidepressant drug exposure in patients with recurrent major depressive disorder. *Neuropsychobiology*, 2009, 59: 227-233.

[62] Sharma, V. Loss of response to antidepressants and subsequent refractoriness: Diagnostic issues in a retrospective case series. *Journal of affective disorders*, 2001, 64: 99-106.

[63] Charlier, C, Pinto, E, Ansseau, M, Plomteux, G. Relationship between clinical effects, serum drug concentration, and concurrent drug interactions in depressed patients treated with citalopram, fluoxetine, clomipramine, paroxetine or venlafaxine. *Human psychopharmacology*, 2000, 15: 453-459.

[64] Byrne, S, Rothschild, AJ. Psychiatrists' responses to failure of maintenance therapy with antidepressants. *Psychiatric services*, 1997, 48: 835-837.

[65] Fava, M, Rappe, SM, Pava, JA, Nierenberg, AA, Alpert, JE, Rosenbaum, JF. Relapse in patients on long-term fluoxetine treatment:

Response to increased fluoxetine dose. *Journal of clinical psychiatry,* 1995, 56: 52-55.

[66] Cain, JW. Poor response to fluoxetine: Underlying depression, serotonergic overstimulation, or a "therapeutic window." *Journal of clinical psychiatry,* 1992, 53: 272-277.

[67] Haddad, P. Do antidepressants have any potential to cause addiction? *Journal of psychopharmacology,* 1999, 13: 300-307.

[68] Bertschy, G, Luxembourger, I, Bizouard, P, Vandel, S, Allers, G, Volmat, R. [Amineptin dependence. Detection of patients at risk. *Report of 8 cases].* Encephale, 1990, 16:405-409.

[69] Perera, I, Lim, L. Amineptine and midazolam dependence. *Singapore medical Journal,* 1998, 39: 129-131.

[70] Kisa, C, Bulbul, DO, Aydemir, C, Goka, E. Is it possible to be dependent to Tianeptine, an antidepressant? A case report. *Progress in neuropsychopharmacology and biological psychiatry,* 2007, 31: 776-778.

[71] Quaglio, G, Schifano, F, Lugoboni, F. Venlafaxine dependence in a patient with a history of alcohol and amineptine misuse. *Addiction,* 2008, 103: 1572-1574.

[72] Vandel, P, Regina, W, Bonin, B, Sechter, D, Bizouard, P. [Abuse of tianeptine. A case report]. *Encephale,* 1999, 25: 672-673.

[73] Saatçioğlu, O, Erim, R, Cakmak, D. [A case of tianeptine abuse]. *Turkish Journal of psychiatry,* 2006, 17: 72-75.

[74] Kim, D, Steinhart, B. Seizures induced by recreational abuse of bupropion tablets via nasal insufflation. *CJEM,* 2010, 12: 158-161.

[75] Langguth, B, Hajak, G, Landgrebe, M, Unglaub, W. Abuse potential of bupropion nasal insufflation: a case report. *Journal of clinical psychopharmacology,* 2009, 29: 618-619.

[76] Vetulani, J. Drug addiction. Part II. Neurobiology of addiction. *Polish Journal of pharmacology,* 2001, 53: 303-317.

[77] Gardner, EL. Addiction and brain reward and antireward pathways. *Advnces in psychosomatic medicine,* 2011, 30: 22-60.

[78] Zawertailo, LA, Busto, UE, Kaplan, HL, Greenblatt, DJ, Sellers, EM. Comparative abuse liability of sertraline, alprazolam and dextroamphetamine in humans. *Journal of clinical psychopharmacology,* 1995, 15: 117-124.

[79] Gold, LH, Balster, RL. Evaluation of nefazodone self-administration in rhesus monkeys. *Drugs and alcohol dependence,* 1991, 28: 241-247.

[80] Oswald, I, Brezinova, V, Dunleavy, DLF. On the slowness of action of tricyclic antidepressant drugs. *British Journal of pychiatry*, 1972, 120: 673-677.

[81] Moreno Brea, MR, Rojas Corrales, O, Gibert-Rahola, J, Micó, JA. [Drug interactions of methadone with CNS-active agents]. *Actas espanolas de psiquiatria*, 1999, 27: 103-110.

[82] Eschalier, A, Ardid, D, Coudore, F. Pharmacological studies of the analgesic effect of antidepressants. *Clinical Neuropharmacology*, 1992, 15: 373A-374A.

[83] Banks, ML, Rice, KC, Negus, SS. Antinociceptive interactions between Mu-opioid receptor agonists and the serotonin uptake inhibitor clomipramine in rhesus monkeys: role of Mu agonist efficacy. *Journal of pharmacology and experimental therapeutics*, 2010, 335: 497-505.

[84] Cohen, MJ, Hanbury, R, Stimmel, B. Abuse of amitriptyline. *JAMA*, 1978, 240: 1372-1373.

[85] Dorman, A, Byrne, P, Talbot, D, O'Connor, J. Misuse of dothiepin. *BMJ*, 1995, 311: 1502.

[86] Darke, S, Ross, J. The use of antidepressants among injecting drug users in Sydney, Australia. *Addiction*, 2000, 95: 407–417.

[87] Peles, E, Schreiber, S, Adelson, M. Tricyclic antidepressants abuse, with or without benzodiazepines abuse, in former heroin addicts currently in methadone maintenance treatment (MMT). *European neuropsychopharmacology*, 2008, 18: 188-193.

[88] Samanin, R, Jori, A, Bernasconi, S, Morpugo, E, Garattini, S. Biochemical and pharmacological studies on amineptine (S 1964) and (+) amphetamine in the rat. *Journal of pharmacy and pharmacology*, 1997, 29: 555-558.

[89] Ponzio, F, Achilli, G, Garattinni, S, Perego, C, Sacchetti, G, Algeri, S. Amineptine: its effects on the dopaminergic system of rats. *Journal of pharmacy and pharmacology*, 1986, 38: 301-303.

[90] Mercuri, NB, Federici, M, Marinelli, S, Bernardi, G. Tranylcypromine, but not moclobemide, prolongs the inhibitory action of dopamine on midbrain dopaminergic neurons: an in vitro electrophysiological study. *Synapse*, 2000, 37: 216-221.

[91] Learned-Coughlin, SM, Bergström, M, Savitcheva, I, Ascher, J, Schmith, VD, Långstrom, B. In vivo activity of bupropion at the human dopamine transporter as measured by positron emission tomography. *Biological psychiatry*, 2003, 54: 800-805.

In: Antidepressants
Editors: L. J. Mígne and J. W. Post

ISBN: 978-1--62081-555-7
© 2012 Nova Science Publishers, Inc.

Chapter 3

ANTIDEPRESSANTS: PHARMACOLOGY, HEALTH EFFECTS AND CONTROVERSY

Preetpal, Susheela Rani, Ashok Kumar Malik, and Jatinder S. Aulakh*

Department of Chemistry,Punjabi University,
Punjab, India

ABSTRACT

"Antidepressant" is the category of drug that acts in a disease specific way to reverse the neuropathological basis of the symptoms of depression. Symptoms of depression include depressed mood, diminished pleasure, change in appetite or weight, alterations in sleep, psychomotor retardation, fatigue, inability to concentrate, indecisiveness, and thoughts of suicide.

This review aim to show the pharmacology, health effects and controversy related to antidepressants. All currently available anti-depressants can be classified into 3 classes: (1) MAOIs, (2) biogenic amine neurotransmitters (3) serotonin type 2A receptor blockers.

Here we considered the antidepressants which are pharmacologically as effective as the WHO claims them to be. Overprescription and misuse of antidepressants is harmful. Over the past decade, the tricyclic

---

* E-mail: malik_chem2002@yahoo.co.uk

antidepressants have been replaced by SSRIs. But it is still controversial whether the newer antidepressants are as effecteive as the older generation compounds. This is also a part of discussion whether antidepressants are helpful in changing the rate of suicide cases and the effect of antidepressants changes with season, nation and gender? Pharmaceutical companies are seeking compounds that can block all the three transporters (the acronym of which is *SNUB* or *super neurotransmitter uptake blocker*). Pharmacogenetics is also helpful treatment of depression. Research has shown that the response to an SSRI is predicted by the genotype of the patient with respect to his or her serotonin transporter.

1. INTRODUCTION

Depression is a medical illness that involves the mind and body. It is also called major depressive disorder and clinical depression. It affects our thinking and behaviour. Depression can lead to a variety of emotional and physical problems. It can cause trouble in doing normal day-to-day activities, and depression may make us feel as if life isn't worth living. Depression is a chronic illness that usually requires long-term treatment, like diabetes or high blood pressure. Most people with depression feel better with psychological counseling, medication or other treatment. According to a publication of the World Health Report 2001, depression will be the world's second leading health problem after heart disease by the year 2020, if calculated by disability adjusted life years (DALYs). Depression may increase the risk of coronary artery disease. The economic effect of depression is also substantial as estimated cost of depression in the United States in 1990 was $44 billion [10]. Surveys by the National Institute of Mental Health shows that about 70 % of the depressed patients don't receive treatment.

An *antidepressant* is a psychiatric medication used to alleviate mood disorders, such as major depression and dysthymia and anxiety disorders such as social anxiety disorder. The term *antidepressant* is sometimes applied to any therapy (e.g., psychotherapy, electro-convulsive therapy, acupuncture) or process (e.g., sleep disruption, increased light levels, regular exercise) found to improve a clinically depressed mood. Many drugs produce an antidepressant effect, but restrictions on their use have caused controversy. Despite of superior efficacy, off-label prescription is always a risk. Symptoms of depression can vary, and one antidepressant may relieve certain symptoms better than another. For example, if your depression symptoms include low energy, an antidepressant that's slightly stimulating may be the best choice. On the other hand, if you have trouble sleeping, an antidepressant that's slightly sedating may be a good option. On October 6, 1966, LSD (League for Spiritual Discovery) [17] was made illegal in the United States and controlled so strictly that not only were possession and recreational use criminalized, but all legal scientific research programs on the drug in the US were shut down as well.

Opioids were used to treat major depression until the late 1950s. Amphetamines were used until the mid 1960s. Use of opioids or amphetamines for depression falls into a legal grey area. Research has only rarely been conducted into the therapeutic potential of opioid derivatives for depression in the past sixty years, whereas amphetamines have found a thriving market for conditions as widely arrayed as attention deficit disorder, narcolepsy, and obesity, and continue to be studied for myriad applications. Both opioids and amphetamines show results within twenty-four to forty-eight hours as they induce therapeutic response very quickly; the therapeutic ratios for both opioids and amphetamines are greater than those of the tricyclic antidepressants. In some of this little, heavily restricted research, the opioid buprenorphine has shown the greatest potential for treating severe, treatment-resistant depression of any known pharmaceutical in a small study that is generally recognized and was published in 1995, but has never been pursued due to the social stigma attached to opioids in addition to that attached to mental illness in America. Most typical antidepressants are usually administered for anywhere from months to years due to delayed onset of action (2–6 weeks). Despite the name, antidepressants are often used controversially, and with a dearth of empirical evidence to support their indication, off-label to treat other conditions, such as anxiety disorders, obsessive compulsive disorder, eating disorders, chronic pain, and some hormone-mediated disorders such as dysmenorrhea. These medications can be used alone or together with anticonvulsants (e.g., Tegretol or Depakote), to treat attention-deficit hyperactivity disorder (ADHD) and substance abuse by addressing underlying depression. Sometimes, antidepressants have also been used to treat snoring and migraines.

Antipsychotics in low doses and benzodiazepines, may be used to manage depression, but they are not antidepressants. An extract of the herb St John's Wort is commonly used as an antidepressant. It is labeled as a dietary supplement in some countries. Inert placebos can have significant antidepressant effects, and so to establish a substance as an "antidepressant" in a clinical trial it is necessary to show superior efficacy to placebo.

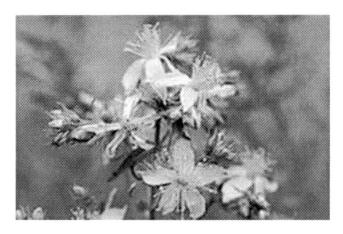

Figure 1. St John's Wort [1].

A review of both published and unpublished trials submitted to the U.S. Food and Drug Administration (FDA) found that the published trials had a 94% success in treating depression while the unpublished literature had below 50% success. Combined, 51% of all studies showed efficacy.

The difference in effect between active placebos and several anti-depressants appeared small and strongly affected by publication bias. Some studies had showed that mirtazapine and venlafaxine may have greater efficacy than other antidepressants in the treatment of severe depression. .

2. HISTORY

Various opiates (via the μ-opioid receptor and κ-opioid receptor) and amphetamines were commonly used as antidepressants until the mid-1950s, when they fell out of favor due to their addictive nature and side-effects [2]. Extracts from the herb St John's Wort have long been used (as a "nerve tonic") to "nerve tonic") to alleviate depression [3].

2.1. Role of Isoniazid and Iproniazid in the History of Antidepressants

In 1951, two people from Sea View Hospital on Staten Island, Irving Selikoff and Edward Robitzek, began clinical trials on two new anti-tuberculosis agents from Hoffman-LaRoche, isoniazid and iproniazid. Only patients with a poor prognosis were initially treated; nevertheless, their condition improved dramatically.

The promise of a cure for tuberculosis in the Sea View Hospital trials was excitedly discussed in the mainstream press. In 1952, learning of the stimulating side-effects of isoniazid, the Cincinnati psychiatrist Max Lurie tried it on his patients. In the following year, he and Harry Salzer reported that isoniazid improved depression in two thirds of their patients and coined the term *antidepressant* to describe its action.

A similar incident took place in Paris, where Jean Delay, head of psychiatry at Sainte-Anne Hospital, found out from his pulmonology colleagues at Cochin Hospital about the side-effects of isoniazid. In 1952, before Lurie and Salzer, Delay, with the resident Jean-Francois Buisson, reported the positive effect of isoniazid on depressed patients. For reasons unrelated to its efficacy, isoniazid as an antidepressant was soon over-shadowed by the more toxic iproniazid, although it remains a mainstay of tuberculosis treatment. The mode of antidepressant action of isoniazid is still unclear. It is speculated that its effect is due to the inhibition of diamine oxidase, coupled with a weak inhibition of monoamine oxidase A.

Another anti-tuberculosis drug tried at the same time by Selikoff and Robitzek, iproniazid, showed a greater "psychostimulant" effect, but more pronounced toxicity. After the publications on isoniazid, papers by Jackson Smith, Gordon Kamman, George Crane, and Frank Ayd appeared, describing the psychiatric applications of iproniazid. Ernst Zeller found iproniazid to be a potent monoamine oxidase inhibitor.

Nevertheless, iproniazid remained relatively obscure until Nathan Kline who were the influential and flamboyant head of research at Rockland State Hospital, began to popularize it in the medical and popular press as a "psychic energizer". Roche put a significant marketing effort behind iproniazid, including promoting its off-label use for depression. Its sales grew massively in the following years, until it was recalled from the market in 1961 due to cases of lethal hepatotoxicity.

2.2. Imipramine

The discovery that a tricyclic ("three ringed") compound had a significant antidepressant effect was first made in 1957 by Roland Kuhn in a Swiss psychiatric hospital. By that time antihistamine derivatives were increasingly used to treat surgical shock and then as psychiatric neuroleptics. In 1955 reserpine was found to be more effective than placebo in alleviating anxious depression, neuroleptics (literally, "to seize the nerves" or "to take hold of nerves") were being developed as antipsycotics and sedatives.

Attempting to improve the effectiveness of chlorpromazine, Kuhn, in conjunction with the Geigy pharmaceutical company, discovered that compound "G 22355" (manufactured and patented in the US in 1951 by Häfliger and Schinder) had a beneficial effect in patients with depression accompanied by mental and motor retardation.

Kuhn first reported his findings on "thymoleptic" (means, "taking hold of the emotions," in contrast with neuroleptics, "taking hold of the nerves") in 1955-56. These gradually became established, resulting in marketing of the first tricyclic antidepressant, imipramine, soon followed by variants.

2.3. Later History

These new drug therapies became prescription drugs in the 1950s and no more than 50 to 100 people per million suffered from the kind of depression that these new drugs would treat. Sopharmaceutical companies were not enthusiastic. Sales through the 1960s remained poor compared to the major tranquilizers (neuroleptics/antipsychotics) and minor tranquilizers (such as benzodiazepines), which were being marketed for different uses. Imipramine remained in common use and numerous successors were introduced. The field of MAO inhibitors remained quiet for many years until "reversible" forms affecting only the MAO-A subtype were introduced, avoiding some of the adverse effects.

Most pharmacologists by the 1960s thought the main therapeutic action of tricyclics was to inhibit norepinephrine reuptake, but it was gradually observed that this action was associated with energizing and motor stimulating effects, while some antidepressant compounds appeared to have differing effects through action on serotonin systems (notably proposed in 1969 by Carlsson and Lindqvist as well as Lapin and Oxenkrug).

Researchers began a process of rational drug design to isolate antihistamine-derived compounds that would selectively target these systems. The first such compound to be patented was zimelidine in 1971, while the first released clinically was indalpine.

Fluoxetine was approved for commercial use by the Food and Drug Administration (United States) in 1988, becoming the first blockbuster SSRI.

Fluoxetine was developed at Eli Lilly and Company in the early 1970s by Bryan Molloy, David Wong and others.

While it had fallen out of favor in most countries through the 19th and 20th centuries, the herb St John's Wort became increasingly popular in Germany, where Hypericum extracts were eventually licensed, packaged and prescribed by doctors. Small-scale efficacy trials were carried out in the 1970s and 1980s, and attention grew in the 1990s following a meta-analysis of these. It remained an over-the-counter drug (OTC) or supplement in most countries and research continued to investigate its neurotransmitter effects and active components, particularly hyperforin [6, 7]

SSRIs became known as "novel antidepressants" along with other newer drugs such as SNRIs and NRIs with various selective effects, such as venlafaxine, duloxetine, nefazodone and mirtazapine [8]

3. CLASSIFICATION OF ANTIDEPRESSANTS

3.1. Functional Classification of Antidepressants

Neurotransmitters are associated with depression, particularly the neurotransmitters serotonin (ser-oh-TOE-nin), norepinephrine (nor-ep-ih-NEF-rin) and dopamine (DOE-puh-mene). Most antidepressants work in depression by affecting these neurotransmitters.

Each type (class) of antidepressant affects these neurotransmitters in slightly different ways. At present, a broad range of structures make up the antidepressant pharmacopoeia, but there are only a few known functional (possibly therapeutic) effects of these compounds. Therefore, a functional classification of antidepressants is more useful than a structural one.

Although not a completely satisfactory strategy, all currently available antidepressants can be classified into 1 of 3 classes: (1) MAOIs, (2) biogenic amine neurotransmitters (serotonin, norepinephrine, and dopamine) reuptake blockers, or (3) serotonin type 2A (5-HT$_{2A}$) receptor blockers.

This functional classification eliminates the confusion in the literature from the incorrect use of terms such as *heterocyclic*, *tricyclic*, and *tetracyclic*. For example, imipramine is both a heterocyclic and a tricyclic antidepressant.

3.2. Types of Antidepressants Depending upon their Structures and Mode of Action

3.2.1. Selective Serotonin Reuptake Inhibitors (SSRIs)

Many doctors start depression treatment by prescribing an SSRI. SSRIs are safe and relieve depression for most people. However, like many antidepressants, they can cause sexual side effects — most commonly failure to achieve orgasm in women and delayed ejaculation in men. SSRIs includes:

a) Citalopram (Celexa)
b) Escitalopram (Lexapro)
c) Fluoxetine (Prozac, Prozac Weekly, Sarafem)
d) Fluvoxamine (Luvox, Luvox CR)
e) Paroxetine (Paxil, Paxil CR, Pexeva)
f) Sertraline (Zoloft)

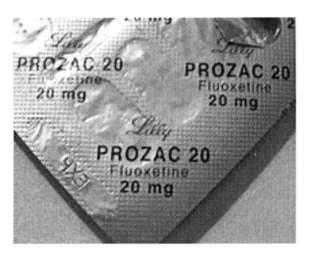

Figure 2. Fluoxetine (Prozac), an SSRI [1].

3.2.2. Serotonin and Norepinephrin Reuptake Inhibitor (SNRIs)

SNRIs include:

a) *Venlafaxine (Effexor XR).* Venlafaxine may work for some people when other antidepressants haven't. It can cause side effects similar to those caused by SSRIs. Venlafaxine can raise blood pressure, and overdose can be dangerous or fatal.

b) *Desvenlafaxine (Pristiq)*. Desvenlafaxine is similar to venlafaxine and causes similar side effects. Studies haven't proven any advantage to desvenlafaxine over venlafaxine, and since venlafaxine is available in a generic form, it's generally a more affordable option.

c) *Duloxetine (Cymbalta)*. In addition to depression, Duloxetine may help in relieving physical pain, but it isn't clear yet whether it works better than other antidepressants for pain relief. Duloxetine can cause a number of side effects. Nausea, dry mouth and constipation are particularly common. People who are heavy drinkers or having liver or kidney problems shouldn't take duloxetine.

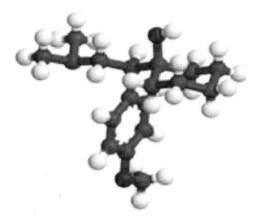

Figure 3. The chemical structure of venlafaxine (Effexor), an SNRI [1].

3.2.3. Atypical Antidepressants

This class of antidepressants is called "atypical" because they don't fit neatly into other categories. Generally, atypical antidepressants cause fewer sexual side effects than other antidepressants do. Atypical antidepressants include:

a) *Bupropion* (Wellbutrin, Wellbutrin SR, Wellbutrin XL) has few sexual side effects. It may also suppress appetite, and it may help you stop smoking if you're trying to quit. People with seizure disorders or who have bulimia or anorexia shouldn't take bupropion.

b) *Trazodone (Oleptro)*. This mild antidepressant is often prescribed as a sleep aid because it can be very sedating.

c) *Mirtazapine* (Remeron, Remeron SolTab). Mirtazapine is also sedating in its effect like trazodone.It may increase lipid levels and cholesterol.

d) *Nefazodone.* This antidepressant is effective, but isn't commonly prescribed because it has been linked to dangerous liver problems.

3.2.4. Tricyclic and Tetracyclic Antidepressants

These older antidepressants are effective, but are usually not a first-choice treatment for depression because of numerous side effects such as dry mouth, constipation, difficulty urinating, sedation, weight gain and sexual side effects. In some cases, a low dose of a cyclic antidepressant may be added to another antidepressant, such as an SSRI, to increase the antidepressant effect. Over-dosing on a cyclic antidepressant can be deadly. These medications are not usually given to older adults or people who have low blood pressure or certain heart problems.

Tricyclic and tetracyclic antidepressants include: *Amitriptyline, Clomipramine* (Anafranil), *Doxepin* (Silenor, Zonalon), *Imipramine* (Tofranil, Tofranil-PM), *Trimipramine* (Surmontil), *Desipramine* (Norpramin), *Nortriptyline* (Pamelor, Aventyl), *Protriptyline* (Vivactil), *Amoxapine, Maprotiline.*

3.2.5. Monoamine Oxidase Inhibitors (MAOIs)

Monoamine oxidase inhibitors are used as a last resort because of numerous bothersome and potentially dangerous serious side effects. However, MAOIs can be effective for some forms of depression when other medications haven't worked. Side effects can include dizziness, dry mouth, upset stomach, difficult urination, twitching muscles, sexual side effects, drowsiness and sleep problems. MAOIs can cause potentially fatal high blood pressure when combined with certain foods and beverages and certain other medications. MAOIs include:

a) Isocarboxazid (Marplan)
b) Phenelzine (Nardil)
c) Tranylcypromine (Parnate)
d) Selegiline (Emsam, Eldepryl, Zelapar)

Emsam is a type of MAOI that you stick on your skin (transdermal patch). It appears to have fewer side effects than MAOIs in pill form have, and with lower dose patches, dietary restrictions may not be needed.

4. PHARMACOTHERAPY FOR DEPRESSION

Antidepressants are given in combination with psychotherapy. If there is mild depression then psychotherapy alone may be of use but some studies have shown that use of antidepressants alongwith some psychotherapy is superior to either treatment alone, specially is case of more severe depression.

4.1. Pharmacology of Antidepressants

a) *Onset of Activity*: After the initiation of treatment, antidepressants shows mood - elevating effects within one – two weeks. Although these drugs shows synaptic effects within hours after the patient ingests the drug. An ideal drug should start work in the same time course as the synaptic effects. All the antidepressants appear to work in the same time course. Drugs take a time period of atleast six weeks to show any change in depression.

Some data suggest that drugs that have actions on both serotonergic and noradrenergic systems ("dual action" compounds) have a quicker onset of action than that of other drugs. However, their efficiency remains almost same.

b) *Elimination Half Life*: Time taken by a drug to eliminate the one half of its amount from the plasma gives us the information about its dosing schedule. Ideal antidepressants should have a half life of about twenty four hours. If a drug has short half life then it reaches the steady state earlier and is eliminated faster than a drug which have longer half life.

Drug which has half life of one day, its steady state is reached after four to five days. Ideally both the parent compound and the active metabolite should have an intermediate half life.

Pharmacokinetic rule based on the elimination half-life is that it takes about 4 to 5 times the elimination half-life to have more than 90% of the drug eliminated from the body after the medication is discontinued. Thus, a drug with an intermediate half-life shortens the time to steady state and for elimination. This knowledge is important when therapy is initiated, when dosages are adjusted, when a medication is discontinued because of an adverse effect, or when one drug is discontinued before another drug is initiated that might cause a drug intraction.

c) *Therapeutic blood levels*: Interindividual variations in the blood levels of an antidepressant with a given dose can be substantial. If a defined therapeutic blood level were known, the dose of the medication could be tailored to the patient to achieve therapeutic effects and avoid adverse effects of antidepressants. Therapeutic drug monitoring may help to avoid toxicity and to increase response rate [21, 22, 23] .

d) *Adverse Effects of Antidepressants*: Adverse effects of antidepressants can be explained by their synaptic effects. Antidepressants affest our body by intracting with the important components of the synapse in the brain. The two most important synaptic effects of antidepressants are:

1) blockade of transport of certain neurotransmitters (norepinephrine, serotonin, and dopamine) back into the nerve ending, and
2) blockade of certain receptors for some neurotransmitters.

Most clinically relevant receptor blockade is at the α_1- adrenergic, dopamine D_2, histamine H_1, muscarinic acetylcholine, and, possibly, 5-HT_{2A} receptors. . Some of these synaptic effects may be required for the therapeutic effects of antidepressants. If so, then antidepressants which are available can never be devoid of adverse effects caused by interactions with neuro-transmitters or their receptors.

Tricyclic antidepressants have effects on cardiac action potentials typical of class IA antiarrhythmics [13], which include drugs such as quinidine and procainamide. Class I antiarrhythmics have been implicated to increase mortality after myocardial infarction, leading to concern about the use of tricyclic antidepressants in patients with cardiovascular disease [14].

This property of tricyclic antidepressants accounts for a serious risk of cardiotoxicity and contributes toward the narrow therapeutic index of tricyclic antidepressants and partly explains the high toxicity of tricyclic anti-depressants and similar compounds with an overdose compared with newer generation compounds (Table 2).

Pharmacodynamic drug interactions are related to the effect of one drug on the mechanism of action of another drug (which the patient is already taking).

Table 1. Functional Classification of Antidepressants [4]

Function	Name of Antidepressant
Dopamine transport blocker Monoamine oxidase inhibitor	Bupropion Tranylcypromine Phenelzine
	Isocarboxazid
Serotonin 5-HT2A receptor blocker	Trazodone Nefazodone
Norepinephrine transport blocker	Mirtazapine Nortriptyline Amoxapine Desipramine Protriptyline Reboxetine*
	Maprotiline Doxepine Amitriptyline Citalopram Clomipramine** Fluoxetine
Serotonin transport blocker	Fluvoxamine**
	Imipramine Paroxetine
	Sertraline
	Trimipramine Venlafaxine

*Not approved for use in the United States.
**Approved for use in the United States for the treatment of obsessive-compulsive disorder.
$5\text{-}HT_{2A}$ = 5-hydroxytryptamine.

Table 2. Relative Toxicity of Antidepressants with Overdose [4]

Relative toxicity with overdose	Name of Antidepressants
	Bupropion Reboxetine Sertraline
	Fluvoxamine
Low	Paroxetine
	Nefazodone
	Mirtazapine
High	Monoamine oxidase
Very high	Amoxapine
	Maprotiline Tricyclic antidepressants

Most of the pharmacodynamic effects of antidepressants relate to their synaptic effects (discussed subsequently). The likelihood of an antidepressant causing a clinically meaningful pharmacodynamic drug interaction is shown in Table 3.

e) *Drug Interactions*: Drug interactions can be divided into two categories: pharmacodynamic and pharmacokinetic that might protect against the development of the serotonergic syndrome.

Table 3. Pharmacodynamic Drug Interactions of Antidepressants [4]

Interaction	Antidepressant
With serotonin selective reuptake inhibitors—lethal	Monoamine oxidase inhibitors
With monoamine oxidase inhibitors—lethal	Citalopram
	Clomipramine
	Fluoxetine
	Fluvoxamine
	Nefazodone*
	Imipramine
	Paroxetine
	Sertraline
	Venlafaxine
With most drugs—little	Bupropion
	Mirtazapine
	Reboxetin

*Nefazodone has some serotonin receptor blocking properties.

Most of the pharmacokinetic drug interactions of antidepressants are related to their inhibitory effects on drug-metabolizing enzymes. Antidepressants inhibit the enzymes of class cytochrome P-450 (CYP). Out of which only three enzymes are of concern- CYP1A2, CYP2D6, and CYP3A4. Nearly all the drugs are metabolized by these 3 enzymes.

Antidepressants that are especially potent inhibitors of these enzymes are fluvoxamine at CYP1A2, paroxetine and fluoxetine at CYP2D6, and nefazodone at CYP3A4. The likelihood of the newer generation antidepressants causing a pharmacokinetic drug interaction is ranked in Table 4.

Table 4. Likelihood of an Antidepressant Causing Pharmacokinetic Drug Interactions at Cytochrome P-450 Enzymes [4]

Liklihood	Name of Antidepressant
Least	Venalafexine
	Citalopram
	Mirtazapine
	Reboxetine
Less	Bupropion
	Sertraline
Most	Fluoxetine
	Fluvoxamine
	Nefazodone
	Paroxetine

Table 5. Possible Therapeutic and Adverse Effects of Transporter and Receptor Blocking Effects of Antidepressant Drugs*[4]

	Possible effects	
	Therapeutic	Adverse
Norepinephrine	Antidepressant	Tremors
transporter		Tachycardia
		Blockade of antihypertensitve effects of guanethidine and guanadel
		Augmentation of pressor effects of sympathomimetic amines
Serotonin transporter	Antidepressant	Gastrointestinal disturbances (including
		weight loss early in treatment, weight gain late in treatment)
		Increase or decrease in anxiety (dose Dependent)
		Sexual dysfunction (including decreased libido)
		Extrapyramidal adverse effects
		Interactions with tryptophan, monoamine
		oxidase inhibitors, and fenfluramine

Table 5. (Continued)

Dopamine D2 receptor	Amelioration of signs	Extrapyramidal movement disorders—dystonia, parkinsonism, akathisia, tardive dyskinesia, rabbit syndrome
	Symptoms of psychosis	Endocrine effects—prolactin elevation (galactorrhea, gynecomastia, menstrual changes, Sexual dysfunction in men)
A1-Adrenoceptors	Unknown	Potentiation of antihypertensive effect of prazosin, terazosin, doxazosin, and labetalol
		Postural hypotension and dizziness
		Reflex tachycardia
Dopamine transporter	Antidepressant	Psychomotor activation
	Antiparkinsonian	Precipitation or aggravation of psychosis
Histamine H1 receptor	Sedation	Sedation
		Drowsiness
		Weight gain
		Potentiation of central depressant drugs
Muscarinic receptor	Antidepressant	Blurred vision
		Attack or exacerbation of narrow-angle glaucoma
		Dry mouth
		Sinus tachycardia
		Constipation
		Urinary retention
		Memory dysfunction

	Possible effects	
	Therapeutic	Adverse
5-HT2A receptor	Antidepressant	
	Reduction of anxiety	
	Promotion of deep sleep	Unknown
	Prophylaxis of migraine	
	headaches	
	Antipsychotic	

*5-HT2A = 5-hydroxytryptamine.

Pharmacokinetic drug interactions are a likely consequence when one drug is combined with another drug, which might inhibit drug-metabolizing enzymes. Additionally, even drugs in the low-risk category might cause a pharmacokinetic drug interaction.

f) *Synaptic Effects of Antidepressants*: Most of the antidepressants show their effect at the level of synapse- the site in the nervous system where one neuron communicates with another neuron or another type of cell (eg, smooth muscle cell). Antidepressants changes the magnitude of the effects of neurotransmitters at these synapses, by blocking uptake of neurotransmitters, blocking certain neuro-transmitter receptors, or inhibiting the mitochondrial enzyme monoamine oxidase.

. Neurotransmitters are the chemicals that neurons use to communicate with one another. Generally these are the small molecules (usually amino acids or their derivatives). Neurotransmitters are released from the nerve ending to bind to specific receptors on the outside surface of cells. Receptors are highly specialized proteins. Each neurotransmitter has at least one unique receptor which binds selectively. There are many examples (eg, for the neuro-transmitter serotonin, which is 5-hydroxytryptamine) of multiple subtypes of receptors for the neurotransmitter. When the chemical messenger binds to its postsynaptic receptor on the receiving neuron, this neuron is changed electrically and biochemically because of the coupling of the neurotransmitter-receptor complex to other components of the membrane in which the receptor resides. Autoreceptors which are present on the cell bodies and terminals, help the neurons in regulating their own activity by feedback mechanisms. 5-HT_{1A} receptor present on the somatodendritic region of the raphe nucleus serotonergic neuron is an example of autoreceptor. Activation of this autoreceptor with the overflow of serotonin inhibits the firing rate of action potentials of this neuron ("negative feedback loop"). Some biogenic amine neurotransmitters are taken back into the nerve ending after release for example norepinephrine, serotonin, and dopamine. This process is called uptake, reuptake, or transport. Transport proteins or transporters , help in the process of reuptake. Overstimulation of receptors in the synapse is also prevented by this transport process. By blocking this transport with a drug we can enhance the neurotransmission early (in the absence of any presynaptic, negative feedback loops). But after a long term treatment adaptive mechanism come into play in which desensitization is followed by down- regulation. Desensitization is the loss of sensitivity of the cell to the neurotransmitter and down – regulation is the loss of the receptor protein from the surface of the cell. As a result, neurotransmission can be diminished or increased if desensitized and down – regulated receptors are inhibitory receptors. Desensitization and down – regulation also explains the reversal of gastrointestinal side effects of SSRIs and therapeutic effects. It also explains the reversal of SSRI appetite – suppressing effects, which can ultimately lead to weight gain late during therapy. A given receptor may or may not show the adaptive mechanism depending on the cell type on which it resides. So, adaptive mechanism of receptors may not occur with all receptors. Antidepressant mirtazapine may cause its therapeutic effects by directly blocking presynaptic α_2-adrenoceptors and some postsynaptic receptors (eg5-HT_{2A}) [15, 16]. Effects of neurotransmitter can be abolished by blocking the receptor with an antagonist. But in case of long – term blockade , another type of things happen because in that case receptor undergoes another type of compensatory change and becomes more sensitive (supersensitive) to the neurotransmitter. This supersensitivity is related to development of tardive dyspinesia after long – term treatment with dopamine D_2 receptor blocking neuroleptics[20] because supersensitivity is accompanied by up -regulation of receptor – related adverse effects of antidepressants.

Some antidepressants inhibit the activity of monoamine oxidase, an enzyme that is important in degradation of catecholamines and serotonin, its inhibition results in an increase in the concentration of neurotransmitter available for release at the synapse because this enzyme is present in mitochondria, which are found in the nerve ending. In addition to this, some antidepressants can block uptake of biogenic amine neurotransmitters and antagonize certain receptors.

4.2. Mechanism of Action of Antidepressants

Most recent theories which explain the mechanism of action of antidepressants focus at the level of gene expression instead of focusing at certain receptors. Serotonin and norepinephrine play important roles in the mechanism of action of antidepressants. All neurons in the brain that synthesize serotonin are located in the raphe nucleus and neurons that synthesize norepinephrine are localized either in the locus coeruleus or in the lateral ventral tegmental fields. Norandrenergic neurons of the raphe nucleus show a reciprocal relationship with each other because these neurons project to one another. Autoreceptors for serotonin or hetreoreceptors for other neurotransmitters are present on the surface of the cell. Neuron synthesizes and release serotonin. All these receptors are thought to span the membrane seven times and couple to protein within the cells to cause the synthesis of second messengers, such as cyclic adenosine monophosphate. Somatodendtric autoreceptors inhibit the rate of firing of action potentials and presynaptic autoreceptors inhibit the synthesis and release of serotonin. Somatodendtric α_1 _ andrenergic heteroreceptors activate the synthesis of neuron on binding norepinephrin whereas presynaptic α_2 – andrenergic heteroreceptor, when activated by norepinephrine inhibit the release of serotonin.

a. Effect of SSRI on Serotonin Receptor: Effect of SSRI on the serotonin varies with short- term and long – term treatment. long-term treatment of animals with an SSRI results in desensitization and down-regulation [25] of serotonergic, somatodendritic, and presynaptic inhibitory autoreceptors that cause (1) an increased firing rate of raphe neurons (somatodendritic autoreceptors), (2) an increased synthesis of serotonin (presynaptic autoreceptors), and (3) an increased release of serotonin (presynaptic autoreceptors).

However in short-term treatment with an SSRI, elevation of serotonin in the synapse is modest because of negative feedback loops that prevent accumulation of excessive amounts of serotonin [25]. In the continued presence of uptake blockade the synaptic levels of serotonin are increased because of removal of negative feedback loops by desensitization and down-regulation of autoreceptors.

However, this theory is not supported by all the animal studies and it has not yet been shown to occur in humans. But studies has shown to that presynaptic 5- HT_{1A} autoreceptors are involved in the feedback of serotonergic neurons has led to the clinical use of antagonists of this receptor in combination with antidepressants to treat depression. In most studies, pindolol was used , which blocks both serotonergic and adrenergic receptors. But these studies conflicting results as some data have been collected by measuring concentrations of brain serotonin receptor by positron emission tomography (PET) study and this data doesn't seem to support the previously explained theories, which are based on animal studies.

For example brain levels of 5-HT_{1A} receptors in depressed patients, researchers found modestly decreased levels in both untreated and treated depressed patients [24] compared to controls. No difference was noted in the concentration of binding sites between responders and nonresponders to antidepressants. Some PET studies have shown thatdepression is associated with an increase or up- regulation of 5- HT_{2A} by measuring the brain levels of 5- HT_{2A} receptors. Thus brain 5- HT_{2A} receptors remain unchanged or decreased in unreacted depressed patients.

b. Blockade of Neurotransmitter Transport by Antidepressants: Most of the antidepressants are more potent at blocking transport of serotonin rather than blocking transport of norepinehrine. SSRIs are more selective in nature and more potent than older compounds at blocking transport of serotonin over norepinehrine, serotonin and dopamine. Reboxetine, is selective for norepinephrine. Bupropion is more selective for blocking transport of dopamine. Citalopram is most selective but selectivity cannot be equated with the potency because selectivity is derived from a ratio of potencies and Paroxetine is most potent blocker of serotonin transport but not as selective as citalopram. Citalopram is only about one tenth as potent as paroxetine at this blockade but citalopran is ten fold more selective or more specific than paroxetine at blocking transport of serotonin.

c. Blockade of Neurotransmitter Receptors by Antidepressants: Tricyclic antidepressants (older compounds) are stronger than newer generation antidepressants at blocking receptors for neurotransmitters. Mirtazepine is relatively potent in binding to the α_2 adrenoceptor. The most potent receptor blocker interaction of antidepressants takes place at histamine H_1 receptor. Histamine is a putative neurotransmitter in the brain. It acts at three types of receptors, histamine H_1, H_2, and H_3. Histamine H_1 receptors are involved in allergic reactions outside the nervous system. Histamine H_2 receptors are present in the brain and are involved with gastric acid secretion. Histamine H_3

affects the presynaptic synthesis and release of of histamine and other neurotransmitters. A topical antipruritic agent doxepin was reported to cause a tricyclic antidepressant overdose in a child with eczema although child never ingested the drug, but it was absorbed through the skin [18, 19].

The next most potent receptor blocking effect is at the muscarinic acetylcholine receptor. These receptors are a type of cholinergic receptors in the brain and are involved with memory and learning. The concentration of drug at the site of action reveal the affinity of drug to cause adverse effects. Serotonin transport blockade causes sexual adverse effects, including anorgasmy and decreased libido. SSRIs can also cause extrapyramidal adverse effects, paranoid reactions, and intense suicidal preoccupation, which may be secondary to akathisia.

Extrapyramidal effects are due to increased synaptic levels of serotonin, but not due to blockade of dopamine receptors as SSRIs are weak at this binding site. Antidepressants may be responsible for orthostatic hypotension and cardiovascular effect. This can lead to dizziness and reflex tachycardia.

Most antidepressant drugs act not only on molecular targets but also on secondary targets leads to side effects. Neuroleptics have potent blocking effects that induce mania in patients. At present there are many variables, which are responsible for the adverse effects and cannot be measured readily. More specifically, we need to know about not only the concentration of drug but also of the neurotransmitter at the target.

The most compound, amoxapine, is a demethylated derivative of neuroleptic loxapine. Some scientists consider amoxapine as an atypical neuroleptic because of its affinity for 5- HT_{2A} receptor relative to its affinity for D_2 receptors. Amoxapine is given to patients with psychotic depressions because of its dopamine receptor blocking property.

In some clinical trials with paroxetine, it has been shown that it causes dry mouth and constipation in the patients which we will discuss in detail further in this chapter in the health effects of antidepressants.

5. Health Effects of Antidepressants

Overprescription and misuse of antidepressants is harmful. Over the past decade, the tricyclic antidepressants have been replaced by SSRIs. But it is still controversial whether the newer antidepressants are as effecteive as the older generation compounds.

One drug is discontinued before another drug is initiated that might cause a drug interaction.

Side effects of antidepressants vary from one medication to another and from person to person. Sexual side effects are a particularly common reason people stop taking an antidepressant. Some antidepressants can cause dangerous reactions when taken with other medications. We can classify its health effects under different cases as follows:

a) *Weight Gain*: Weight gain is a possible side effect of nearly all antidepressants. However, each person responds to an antidepressant differently. Some people gain weight when taking a certain anti-depressant while others don't. Generally speaking, some anti-depressants seem more likely to cause weight gain than do others.

These include:

1) Tricyclic antidepressants such as amitriptyline, imipramine (Tofranil), and doxepin (Sinequan)
2) Monoamine oxidase inhibitors (MAOIs) such as: tranylcypromine (Parnate), isocarboxazid (Marplan) and phenelzine (Nardil), Paroxetine (Paxil), Mirtazapine (Remeron) and Trazodone.

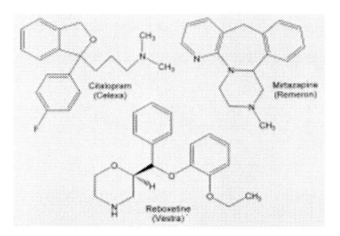

Figure 4. Some Newer Generation Antidepressants [4].

Some antidepressants that may be less likely to cause weight gain include:

1) Venlafaxine (Effexor)
2) Bupropion (Wellbutrin)
3) Selective serotonin reuptake inhibitors (SSRIs) other than paroxetine (Paxil) — fluoxetine (Prozac), sertraline (Zoloft), citalopram (Celexa) and escitalopram (Lexapro)

While some people gain weight after starting an antidepressant, the antidepressant isn't always a direct cause. There are many factors that can work together to contribute to weight gain during antidepressant therapy. For example:

1) Overeating as a result of depression can cause weight gain.
2) Some people lose weight as part of their depression. In turn, an improved appetite associated with improved mood may result in increased weight.
3) Adults generally tend to gain weight each year, regardless of the medications they take. Getting regular exercise and watching what you eat will help you maintain a healthy weight whether you take an antidepressant or not.

b) *If the Person Has Some Particular Symptoms*: Symptoms of depression can vary, and one antidepressant may relieve certain symptoms better than another. For example, if a patient's depression symptoms include low energy, an antidepressant that's slightly stimulating may be the best choice. On the other hand, if patient has trouble sleeping, an antidepressant that's slightly sedating may be a good option.

c) *Some Other Possible Side Effects of Antidepressants:* Side effects of antidepressants vary from one medication to another and from person to person. Bothersome side effects can make it difficult to stick with treatment. Sexual side effects are a particularly common reason due to which people stop taking an antidepressant.

d) *Whether It Worked for a Close Relative:* How a medication worked for a first-degree relative, such as a parent or sibling, can indicate how well it might work for you. It may have side effects which vary from person to person.

e) *Interaction with Other Medications:* Some antidepressants can cause dangerous reactions when taken with other medications.

f) *Whether the Lady is Pregnant or Breast-Feeding:* Many antidepressants may not be safe for your baby when taken during pregnancy or later when you're breast-feeding. Work with your doctor to find the best way to manage your depression when you're expecting.

g) *Some Other Health Conditions of Person:* Some antidepressants may cause problems if you have certain mental or physical health conditions. On the other hand, certain antidepressants may help treat other physical or mental health conditions along with depression. For example, bupropion (Wellbutrin, Wellbutrin SR, Wellbutrin XL) may relieve symptoms of both attention-deficit/hyperactivity disorder (ADHD) and depression.

h) *Some Common Antidepressant Side Effects Are:* Dry mouth, Headache, Dizziness, Nausea, Insomnia, Sexual dysfunction, Weight gain, increased appetite.

7. CONTROVERSY RELATED TO ANTIDEPRESSANTS

It is a part of controversy that whether antidepressants are pharmacologically as effective as the WHO claims them to be? Moreover it is also controversial that whether the newer antidepressants are more or less efficacious than the older generation antidepressants, especially in case of severe depression [11, 12].

Antidepressants when used in the paediatric patients has been linked with the risk of suicidal behaviours [9]. Some data collected by the recent studies on the antidepressants has shown that newer generation compounds offer clear advantages over the tricyclic antidepressants and other older generation compounds. Pharmaceutical companies are seeking compounds that can block all 3 transporters (the acronym of which is *SNUB* or *super neurotransmitter uptake blocker*). But whether they are safe for use patients is still under investigations.

7.1. Recent in Antidepressants

Escitalopram (Lexapro) is a prescription drug commonly used to treat depression and generalized anxiety disorder. Breast tenderness isn't among the published Lexapro side effects [5]. Lexapro may interfere with the normal processing of prolactin — a hormone that affects breast tissue. It's possible that this could lead to breast tenderness. Breast pain has been documented as a rare side effect of other antidepressants, including citalopram (Celexa), sertraline (Zoloft), venlafaxine (Effexor) and mirtazapine (Remeron). Some medications other than antidepressants also have been linked to breast tenderness.

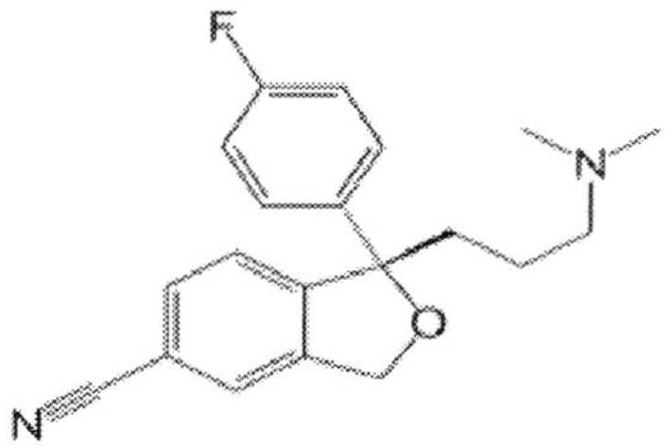

Figure 5. Structural formula of the SSRI escitalopram, in its free base form [1].

7.2. Pristiq (desvenlafaxine)

Pristiq (desvenlafaxine) was approved by the FDA in February of 2008 for the treatment of major depressive disorder in adults [5]. Pristiq works by preventing the reuptake of the serotonin and norepinephrine in the brain.

We know that certain neurotransmitters such as norepinephrine, serotonin and dopamine are not in proper balance when a person is depressed. Like many antidepressants, Pristiq can have side effects, which may include: Nausea, Dizziness, Trouble sleeping, Hyperhidrosis (increased sweating), Constipation, Fatigue, Decreased appetite, Anxiety, Sexual dysfunction in men. But if patient have been diagnosed with depression, Pristiq might be a good option if other medications haven't worked well.

7.3. Lithium Medication [5]

Lithium medication can be used together with other antidepressants to make them more effective. Those taking lithium need to have their blood tested periodically. Possible lithium medication side effects include: Increased urination, Tremors or shaking, Dulling of one's thinking, Nausea, Sedation, Kidney and thyroid disease .Lithium can interact with some medications, and not everyone is a candidate for lithium therapy. Talk with your health care provider for additional information, and share with the group if you've had success with lithium.

7.4. Electroconvulsive Therapy (ECT)

Many people with depression need only a good therapist. Some people need medication. But for others, if both of these therapies are not working well then the answer may be electroconvulsive therapy, or ECT. Here in the Figure 6 a patient is shown who is getting treatment with the ECT.

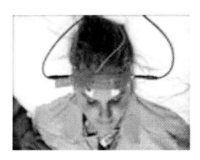

Figure 6. A patient undergoing ECT [5]

REFERENCES

[1]   http://en.wikipedia.org/wiki/Antidepressant.

[2]   Weber, MM; Emrich, HM (July 1988). "Current and Historical Concepts of Opiate Treatment in Psychiatric Disorders". *International Clinical Psychopharmacology* (Lippincott Williams and Wilkins) 3 (3) 255–66. doi:10.1097/00004850-198807000-00007. PMID 3153713. http://journals.lww.com/intclinpsychopharm/ Abstract/1988/07000/Current_and_Historical_Concepts_of_Opiate.7.asp x. Retrieved 2009-05-28.

[3]   Czygan, FC (8 May 2003). "Kulturgeschichte und Mystik des Johanniskrauts: Vom 2500 Jahre alten Apotropaikum zum aktuellen Antidepressivum" (in German). *Pharmazie in unserer Zeit* (Weinheim: WILEY-VCH Verlag) 32 (3): 184–190. doi:10.1002/pauz.200390062. PMID 12784538.

[4]   Review on Pharmacology of Antidepressants, Elliott Richelson, MD, *Mayo Clin Proc.* 2001;76:511-527.

[5]   http://www.mayoclinic.com.

[6]   Müller WE (February 2003). "Current St John's wort research from mode of action to clinical efficacy". *Pharmacol. Res.* 47 (2): 101–9.

doi:10.1016/S1043-6618(02)00266-9. PMID12543057.
http://linkinghub.elsevier.com/retrieve/pii/S1043661802002669.

[7]   Nathan PJ (March 2001). "Hypericum perforatum (St John's Wort): a non-selective reuptake inhibitor? A review of the recent advances in its pharmacology". *J. Psychopharmacol. (Oxford)* 15 (1): 47–54. doi:10.1177/026988110101500109.PMID 11277608.http://jop.sagepub.com/cgi/pmidlookup?view=longandpmid=11277608.

[8]   Freeman, H (1996). "Tolerability and safety of novel antidepressants". *European Psychiatry* 11: 206s. doi:10.1016/0924-9338(96)88597-X.

[9]   Tamar D. Wohlfarth , Barbara J. van Zwieten , Frits J. Lekkerkerker , Christine C. Gispen-de Wied a, Jerry R. Ruis , Andre J.A. Elferink , Jitschak G. Storosum "Antidepressants use in children and adolescents and the risk of suicide". *European Neuropsychopharmacology (2006) 16, 79—83*.

[10] .Greenberg PE, Stiglin LE, Finkelstein SN, Berndt ER. The economic burden of depression in 1990. *J. Clin. Psychiatry*. 1993;54: 405-418.

[11] Steffens DC, Krishnan KR, Helms MJ. Are SSRIs better than TCAs? comparison of SSRIs and TCAs: a meta-analysis. *DepressAnxiety*. 1997;6:10-18.

[12] Anderson IM. Selective serotonin reuptake inhibitors versus tricyclic antidepressants: a meta-analysis of efficacy and tolerability. *J. Affect. Disord*. 2000;58:19-36.

[13] Glassman AH. Cardiovascular effects of antidepressant drugs: updated. *Int. Clin. Psychopharmacol*. 1998;13(suppl 5):S25-S30. 53.

[14] Roose SP, Glassman AH. Antidepressant choice in the patient,with cardiac disease: lessons from the Cardiac Arrhythmia Suppression Trial (CAST) studies. *J. Clin. Psychiatry*. 1994;55(supplA):83-87.

[15] de Boer TH, Maura G, Raiteri M, de Vos CJ, Wieringa J, Pinder RM. Neurochemical and autonomic pharmacological profiles of the 6-aza-analogue of mianserin, Org 3770 and its enantiomers. *Neuropharmacology*. 1988;27:399-408.

[16] Haddjeri N, Blier P, de Montigny C. Effect of the alpha-2 adrenoceptor antagonist mirtazapine on the 5-hydroxytryptamine system in the rat brain. *J. Pharmacol. Exp. Ther*. 1996;277:861- 871.

[17] En.wikipedia.org/wiki/league for spiritual discovery.

[18] Drake LA, Fallon JD, Sober A, Doxepin Study Group. Relief of pruritus in patients with atopic dermatitis after treatment with topical doxepin cream. *J. Am. Acad. Dermatol*. 1994;31:613-616.

[19] Drake LA, Cohen L, Gillies R, et al. Pharmacokinetics of doxepin in subjects with pruritic atopic dermatitis. *J. Am. Acad. Dermatol.* 1999;41(2, pt 1):209-214.

[20] Tarsy D, Baldessarini RJ..The pathophysiologic basis of tardivedyskinesia. *Biol. Psychiatry.* 1977;12:431-450.

[21] Lundmark J, Reis M, Bengtsson F. Therapeutic drug monitoringof sertraline: variability factors as displayed in a clinical setting. *Ther. Drug. Monit.* 2000;22:446-454.

[22] Charlier C, Pinto E, Ansseau M, Plomteux G. Relationship between clinical effects, serum drug concentration, and concurrent drug interactions in depressed patients treated with citalopram, fluoxetine, clomipramine, paroxetine or venlafaxine. *Hum. Psychopharmacol.* 2000;15:453-459.

[23] Burke MJ, Preskorn SH. Therapeutic drug monitoring of antidepressants:cost implications and relevance to clinical practice.*Clin. Pharmacokinet.* 1999;37:147-165.

[24] Sargent PA, Kjaer KH, Bench CJ, et al. Brain serotonin1A receptor binding measured by positron emission tomography with [11C] WAY-100635: effects of depression and antidepressant treatment. *Arch. Gen. Psychiatry.* 2000;57:174-180.

[25] Briley M, Moret C. Neurobiological mechanisms involved in antidepressant therapies. *Clin. Neuropharmacol.* 1993;16:387- 400.

In: Antidepressants
Editors: L. J. Mígne and J. W. Post

ISBN: 978-1--62081-555-7
© 2012 Nova Science Publishers, Inc.

Chapter 4

IMMUNOMODULATORY ACTION OF FLUOXETINE IN NORMAL AND IN PATHOLOGICAL CONDITIONS: CONTROVERSIES REGARDING MALIGNANT PROCESSES

Maximiliano Rapanelli and Luciana Romina Frick[*]

IBYME-CONICET, Vuelta de Obligado,
Buenos Aires, Argentina

ABSTRACT

Antidepressants are used to alleviate mood disorders, such as major depression, dysthymia and anxiety. Among these drugs, selective serotonin reuptake inhibitors such as fluoxetine, act on neuronal cells by targeting the serotonin transporter prolonging the availability of this neurotransmitter on the synaptic space. In the past years, controversial evidences indicate that antidepressants can modulate non-neuronal cell types. Contradictory data indicate both stimulatory and inhibitory effects of antidepressants in immune cells as well as in tumor cells. First, antidepressants are able to reverse the alterations of the immune system observed in humans suffering depression as well as in animal models of

---

[*] Corresponding Author: IBYME-CONICET, Vuelta de Obligado 2490 (C1428ADN), Buenos Aires, Argentina, Tel: 5411 4783 2869 ext 235, E-mail: luciana.frick@conicet.gov.ar

stress. However, fluoxetine also has an effect per se on the immune cells in physiological conditions. Systemic and in vitro fluoxetine administration has been shown to both enhance and inhibit the immune function. The modulatory effect of fluoxetine on the immune function appears to depend on: a) the dose of antidepressant tested and b) the degree of lymphocyte activation. At least in part, this effect is dependent of serotonin reuptake. However, novel pathways that are in part independent of the fluoxetine action on the serotonin transporter are starting to emerge. Interestingly, several antidepressants induce apoptosis in certain kinds of tumors, but also stimulate proliferation on other cancer types. Fluoxetine is one of the most studied antidepressant in this scenario, and was found to affect tumor progression by specific and compensatory mechanisms, some of them seem to be mediated by its action upon the central nervous system, but others are executed directly on peripheral cells.

A BRIEF INTRODUCTION TO DEPRESSION, IMMUNITY AND FLUOXETINE

Fluoxetine is a widely used antidepressant which belongs to the family of selective serotonin reuptake inhibitors. At the central nervous system, this drug increases the extracellular level of the neurotransmitter serotonin by inhibiting its reuptake into the presynaptic neuron, thus increasing the level of serotonin in the synaptic cleft available to bind to the postsynaptic receptor. Fluoxetine is prescribed for the treatment of major depression (including pediatric depression), obsessive-compulsive disorder (in both adult and pediatric populations), bulimia nervosa, panic disorder and premenstrual dysphoric disorder. Depression has been associated with impairments of the immune function, and fluoxetine treatment was found to counteract these negative effects on immunity. In patients with major depression, prolonged fluoxetine treatment reverses the impairment of natural killer (NK) cells activity (Frank et al., 1999). In addition, circulating levels of Interleukin (IL)-12 and the content of serotonin in the lymphocytes from depressed patients are restored by fluoxetine (Lee and Kim, 2006; Lima and Urbina, 2002). This antidepressant treatment also normalized CD16/56 and CD45 values after 6 weeks (Başterzi et al., 2010). However, epidemiological studies provided limited evidence regarding the role of antidepressant on immunity. In this scenario, animal models of psychiatric disorders simulated by chronic exposure to stress are useful tools to unravel this possibility.

FLUOXETINE-INDUCED REVERSION
OF NEGATIVE EFFECTS OF STRESS

Fluoxetine was proven to counteract the detrimental effects of stress in the immune system of rodents. For example after prolonged exposure to auditory stress, NK cell activity is reduced and fluoxetine is able to restore normal values of said activity in a dose-dependent manner (Nuñez et al., 2006). The same effect is observed for cytotoxic activity of T lymphocytes, total counts of peripheral blood lymphocytes, thymus weight, and phagocytic activity of macrophages (Freire-Garabal et al., 1997, 2002; Nuñez et al., 2006). Proliferation of splenocytes is also restored by fluoxetine treatment after the reduction caused by defeat stress (Beitia et al., 2005). In addition, exposure to chronic mild stress induces several effects on the immune system, including reduction of T cell proliferation, increased B cell proliferation, alteration of cAMP and cGMP responses, as well as beta-adrenergic and muscarinic receptors; all of which are reversed by fluoxetine administration (Edgar et al., 2002). Finally, chronic restraint stress in mice causes a general depression of T cell mediated immunity, namely mitogen-induced proliferation, $CD4^+$ total count, and T_H1 cytokine expression (Frick et al., 2009a). Systemic administration of fluoxetine counteracts the negative effects of stress, but interestingly in vitro treatment of "stressed" lymphocytes with fluoxetine is able to reverse the impairment of T cell proliferation by a direct action (Frick et al., 2009b). Similarly, fluoxetine attenuates the basal overactivation of T lymphocytes isolated from depressed patients reinforcing the possibility of a direct antidepressant action (Fazzino et al., 2008). Nevertheless, in normal subjects (not exposed to stress), controversial results were found, some groups found no effects (Freire-Garabal et al., 1997, 2002; Nuñez et al., 2006) whereas other groups found both stimulatory and inhibitory effects of fluoxetine on the immune function, as discussed below.

INTRINSEC EFFECTS OF FLUOXETINE
ON IMMUNE FUNCTION

In healthy mice, it was described that acute but not chronic fluoxetine administration decreases mitogen-induced T lymphocyte proliferation and NK cell cytolytic activity, due to the elevation of extracellular serotonin levels following reuptake inhibition (Pellegrino and Bayer, 2000). Both effects involve the participation of the central nervous system, and the indirect activation of serotonin receptors 5-HT$_2$ was also shown (Pellegrino and Bayer, 1998, 2002). Conversely, prolonged administration of fluoxetine, when it is taken orally, has been shown to enhance T cell proliferation in mice, which is accompanied by increments of IL-2, Interferon (IFN)-γ and Tumor Necrosis Factor (TNF)-α (Frick et al., 2008, 2009b). Moreover, prolonged fluoxetine administration in mice stimulates the proliferative activity of splenocytes and suppresses their ability to secrete the anti-inflammatory cytokine IL-4 (Kubera et al., 2000).

DIRECT ACTION OF FLUOXETINE UPON LYMPHOID CELLS

Interestingly, certain non-neuronal cells express monoamine transporters and receptors; therefore are potential targets of antidepressants. For instance, this is the case of T and B lymphocytes as well as NK cells (Gordon and Barnes, 2003).

In vitro studies performed with isolated lymphoid cells demonstrated that fluoxetine is able to exert certain effects in a direct manner without the participation of the central nervous system. For example, fluoxetine increases the cytotoxic activity of human NK cells in vitro (Frank et al., 1999). Fluoxetine suppresses the ability of dendritic cells to present bacterial antigens to T cells, and the resulting T-cell proliferation, probably due to diminished expression of costimulatory molecules (Branco-de-Almeida et al., 2011). High doses of fluoxetine also affect neutrophil phagocytosis and oxidative burst (Ploppa et al., 2008)..Additionally, low concentrations of fluoxetine (10^{-5} M) inhibit priming but not activation of human polymorphonuclear neutrophils. Instead, at higher concentrations (10^{-4} M), fluoxetine exerts a cytotoxic effects on these cells (Strümper et al., 2003).

Interestingly, fluoxetine exerts a dual effect upon in vitro T cell proliferation, depending on the degree of lymphocyte activation: at optimal concentration concanavalin, fluoxetine has an inhibitory effect on cellular proliferation, whereas at submitogenic concentrations, fluoxetine stimulated the lymphocyte reactivity (Edgar et al., 1998, 1999). These effects are also dependent on fluoxetine concentrations: high doses are toxic whereas low doses are stimulatory. A similar effect was observed for B cell proliferation induced by anti-immunoglobulin M antibodies (Genaro et al., 2000).

Fluoxetine modulation of T cell proliferation is thought to be exerted through protein kinase C (PKC) and protein kinase A (PKA) involving cAMP and Ca^{2+} mobilization (Edgar et al., 1998, 1999).

It is worth noting that the toxic effect of antidepressant on neutrophils and T cells is observed only with high doses, i.e. millimolar concentrations of fluoxetine (Frick et al., 2009b; Ploppa et al., 2008; Strümper et al., 2003). Taking into account these evidences, it would be plausible that antidepressants have a stimulatory effect on immune cells at physiologically relevant concentrations, and that inhibitory effects observed for high doses of antidepressants could be due only to toxic actions. This dual effect also may be influenced by the immunological status of the individual, more specifically by the microbial or tumoral challenges, thus leading to the controversial results observed by different groups.

SEROTONIN-INDEPENDENT MODULATION OF IMMUNE CELLS

At least in part, the effects of fluoxetine on immune cells described above are dependent of serotonin reuptake, as it is expected. However, novel pathways that are in part independent of the fluoxetine action on the serotonin transporter (SERT) are starting to emerge.

It was recently demonstrated that Fluoxetine suppresses the ability of dendritic cells (DCs) to present bacterial antigens to T cells, and the resulting T-cell proliferation, in a serotonin transporter/serotonin (SERT/5-HT)-independent manner (Branco-de-Almeida et al., 2011). In addition, the effects of fluoxetine upon T-cell proliferation in vitro are in part independent of its ability to elevate serotonin extracellular levels (Frick et al., 2008, 2009b). Moreover, high doses (10-50 microM) of fluoxetine inhibit IFN-γ production by T cells, but this effect is proposed to be unrelated to inhibition of monoamine reuptake (Diamond et al., 2006). The novel molecular target of fluoxetine has not been indentified yet.

FLUOXETINE TREATMENT IN CANCER PATIENTS

Fluoxetine, among other antidepressants, is prescribed to treat depressive symptoms in patients with cancer (Fisch et al., 2003; Holland et al., 1998). The use of fluoxetine for 6 months results in an improvement in quality of life, a higher completion of adjuvant treatment (chemotherapy, hormonal therapy, chemotherapy plus hormonal therapy), and a reduction in depressive symptoms (Navari et al., 2008). Moreover, fluoxetine is prescribed to breast carcinoma survivors to treat hot-flashes (Loprinzi et al., 2002; Mariani et al., 2005).

It was suggested that antidepressants could initiate and/or inhibit cancer, but epidemiological studies are controversial. For example, fluoxetine was reported to be both a tumour promoter and an antineoplastic agent (Steingart and Cotterchio, 1995). In fact, Lawlor and colleagues (2003) suggested that epidemiologic evidence available was insufficient to support an association between antidepressant use and breast cancer. A link between fluoxetine and testicular cancer was suggested although not proved (Friedman et al., 2009). Moreover, fluoxetine concomitant treatment may result in the loss of efficacy of certain antineoplasic drugs such as tamoxifen or higher toxicity (Miguel and Albuquerque, 2011).

Conversely, antidepressants were also proposed to be involved in the development of certain types of cancer. The susceptibility to develop cutaneous pseudolymphoma was associated with fluoxetine therapy (Crowson and Magro, 1995). A similar finding was observed for male breast cancer (Wallace et al., 2001). Once again, animal models provided more consistent and robust information on this topic.

EFFECTS OF FLUOXETINE ON TUMOR PROGRESSION

Fluoxetine was found to suppress cell division in chemically-induced colonic tumors in rats, and to retard the growth of human colonic tumor lines propagated as xenografts in immune-deprived mice (Tutton and Barkla, 1982). In addition, fluoxetine inhibits the proliferation of human prostate carcinoma cell lines in vitro and growing in nude mice (Abdul et al., 1995). Fluoxetine also increases volume doubling times of human bronchogenic carcinoma in xenografted mice (Sheehan et al., 1996). In vitro, fluoxetine induces cytotoxicity in human carcinoma HT29 cells (Arimochi and Morita, 2006). More recently, Stepulak and colleagues (2008) demonstrated a growth inhibitory effect of fluoxetine in a variety of tumor types, including in neuroblastoma, medulloblastoma/rhabdomyosarcoma, astrocytoma, lung, colon, and breast cancer.

Several tumor lines undergo apoptosis after fluoxetine treatment in vitro, namely glioma, neuroblastoma, Burkitt lymphoma, ovarian carcinoma (Lee et al. 2010; Levkovitz et al., 2005; Serafeim et al., 2003; Spanová et al., 1997). Interestingly, fluoxetine was also found to induce autophagic cell death in a lymphoma line resistant to apoptosis (Cloonan and Williams, 2011).

Another interesting finding is that Fluoxetine inhibits multidrug resistance (MDR) extrusion pumps and enhances responses to chemotherapy in syngeneic and in human xenograft mouse tumor models (Peer et al., 2004). Furthermore, combinations of fluoxetine with chemotherapeutic drugs such as doxorubicin enhance therapeutic responses to treatment resistant colon cancer caused by MDR (Argov et al., 2009).

Instead in the case of B16F10 melanoma cells and C3 fibrosarcoma cells, Fluoxetine increases proliferation both in vivo and in vitro (Brandes et al., 1992). However, Volpe and coworkers showed that fluoxetine has no effect on B16F10 cells at optimal or suboptimal culture conditions, but inhibits their growth at concentrations above 5 microM along with significant suppression of DNA synthesis in B16F10 and C3 cells at 30 microM (Volpe et al., 2003).

Finally, a recent work demonstrated that fluoxetine has potent selective antiproliferative effects against Burkitt lymphoma independently of the serotonin transporter (Cloonan et al., 2010). This finding provides further evidence on the existence of an alternative pathway of action that is not related to monoamine reuptake, as discussed previously.

INVOLVEMENT OF FLUOXETINE IN REVERSION OF STRESS-INDUCED CANCER PROGRESSION

Taking together the evidences listed above, it seems plausible that fluoxetine (and other antidepressants) can counteract the detrimental impact of stress in cancer progression. In this sense, Freire-Garabal and colleagues (1998) described that fluoxetine is able to reverse the negative effects of the stress caused by a surgery of rats carrying Walker 256 carcinosarcoma cells. In addition, prolonged fluoxetine administration counteracts the negative effects of chronic stress on cancer progression in a lymphoma model (Figure 1).

Although there are not abundant evidences on the effects of fluoxetine in particular, other antidepressants have been studied providing a little extension of these results. Nefazodone, a serotonin and norepinephrine reuptake inhibitor and 5-HT$_{2A}$ receptor antagonist antidepressant, reduces tumor appearance, metastasis and survival of chronically stressed animals (Freire-Garabal et al., 2004). In addition, the tryciclic antidepressant impipramine attenuates the facilitation of tumor growth observed in rats subjected to chronic variable stress (Basso et al., 1992).

It is important to establish a link between antidepressants, cancer and immunity. For instance, Kubera et al. (2009). found an association between B16F10 melanoma growth and the production of IL-6, IL-10 and IL-12p40 in fluoxetine-treated mice that were not subjected to a stressor. Inhibition of lymphoma growth by fluoxetine administration is accompanied by increased IFN-γ and TNF-α levels as well as augmented circulating CD8[+] T lymphocytes (Frick et al. 2011). Instead, chronic stress reduces both cytokines and CD4[+] T cells therefore enhancing lymphoma progression (Frick et al., 2009a).

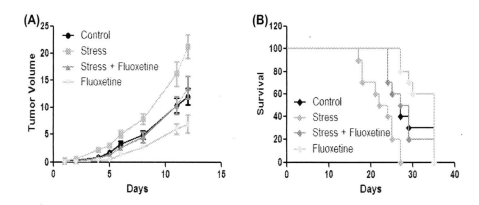

Figure 1. Combined effects of chronic stress and fluoxetine on tumor evolution of the LBC lymphoma cell line. Female BALB/c mice were subjected to chronic restraint stress (for full details of the model, see Frick et al., 2009a), treated with 15mg/kg of oral fluoxetine, or both. All animals were subcutaneously injected with 1 x 10[6] LBC cells to obtain solid tumors. The lymphoma line is described in Frick et al., 2008. (A) *Tumor growth.* Lenght (L) and Width (W) of each tumor were measured and used to calculate the Volume (V) = π/6 x L x W². Means ± SEM are shown (*n* = 10 mice per group). (B) *Survival.* Kaplan-Meier curves show the percentage of survival after tumor injection.

Table 1. Combined effects of chronic stress and fluoxetine on antitumor immunity in lymphoma bearing mice. Cytokine expression in the lymph nodes of the animals subjected to the treatments decribed above was determined by real time PCR and normalized to β-actin. The total events of distinct lymphocyte subpopulations were determined by flow cytometry. For full details of immunity analysis on tumor bearing animals, see Frick et al., 2011.

	Control	Stress	Stress + Fluoxetine	Fluoxetine
IFN-γ expression	25.67 ± 5.26	2.94 ± 0.36 (↓)	29.79 ± 5.05	63.43 ± 3.28 (↑)
TNF-α expression	5.62 ± 0.63	1.51 ± 0.17 (↓)	4.43 ± 0.53	17.87 ± 2.98 (↑)
CD4$^+$ T cells	9.01 ± 0.35	5.28 ± 0.28 (↓)	8.05 ± 0.29	8.77 ± 0.30
CD8$^+$ T cells	2.35 ± 0.24	2.44 ± 0.17	2.74 ± 0.19	3.02 ± 0.23 (↑)

Interestingly, the combination of stress and antidepressant revealed the existence of specific and compensatory mechanisms (see also Frick et al., 2009b). Fluoxetine increases IFN-γ and TNF-α production per se, whereas chronic stress results in the reduction of both cytokines. When both treatments were combined, a compensatory effect was observed, i.e., intermediate cytokine levels were achieved (Table 1).

Chronic stress also resulted in a reduction of CD4$^+$ T cells, and this effect is reversed by fluoxetine administration. Surprisingly, fluoxetine does not have an effect per se on CD4$^+$ subpopulation. With respect to CD8$^+$ T cells, this population is not affected by stress but fluoxetine is able to increase its circulating levels. Therefore, specific effects of fluoxetine were identified (Table 1).

Taking together the results, it is plausible that fluoxetine could inhibit tumor progression by selectively increasing cytotoxic CD8$^+$cells, as it was recently described by Fazzino et al. (2009). On the contrary, stress could promote tumor growth by differentially inducing apoptosis in CD4$^+$ T lymphocytes, in particular T_H1 cells.

This hypothesis, that seems unlikely, is supported by the pioneer work of Toscano et al. (2007), who demonstrated that in pathological conditions certain types of T lymphocytes characterized by their patterns of cytokines: T_H1 and T_H17, display an enhanced susceptibility to cell death compared with other the other type: T_H2 cells.

CONCLUSION

Fluoxetine is undoubtedly involved in the modulation of the immune system and the regulation of cancer progression. The resulting effect will depend on:

1) The degree of T lymphocyte activation
2) The dose of antidepressant tested
3) The type of tumor cell

The mechanisms of action of fluoxetine can be:

1) Serotonin-dependent or independent
2) Direct (on peripheral cells) or indirect (mediated by the nervous system)

This differential action can explain the controversial results observed in preclinical and epidemiological studies. Therefore, fluoxetine could be either beneficial or detrimental when prescribed to patients suffering depression and/or cancer. It is necessary to take this information into account to avoid potential damaging effects of fluoxetine administration as well as to take advantage of its positive action depending of the factors listed above. Personalized treatments according to the individual situation of each patient are encouraged.

REFERENCES

Abdul M, Logothetis CJ, Hoosein NM. Growth-inhibitory effects of serotonin uptake inhibitors on human prostate carcinoma cell lines. *J. Urol.* 1995 Jul;154(1):247-50.

Argov M, Kashi R, Peer D, Margalit R. Treatment of resistant human colon cancer xenografts by a fluoxetine-doxorubicin combination enhances therapeutic responses comparable to an aggressive bevacizumab regimen. *Cancer Lett.* 2009 Feb 8;274(1):118-25.

Arimochi H, Morita K. Characterization of cytotoxic actions of tricyclic antidepressants on human HT29 colon carcinoma cells. *Eur. J. Pharmacol.* 2006 Jul 10;541(1-2):17-23.

Basso AM, Depiante-Depaoli M, Molina VA. Chronic variable stress facilitates tumoral growth: reversal by imipramine administration. *Life Sci.* 1992;50(23):1789-96.

Başterzi AD, Yazici K, Buturak V, Cimen B, Yazici A, Eskandari G, Tot Acar S, Taşdelen B. Effects of venlafaxine and fluoxetine on lymphocyte subsets in patients with major depressive disorder: a flow cytometric analysis. *Prog. Neuropsychopharmacol. Biol. Psychiatry.* 2010 Feb 1;34(1):70-5.

Beitia G, Garmendia L, Azpiroz A, Vegas O, Brain PF, Arregi A. Time-dependent behavioral, neurochemical, and immune consequences of repeated experiences of social defeat stress in male mice and the ameliorative effects of fluoxetine. *Brain Behav. Immun.* 2005 Nov;19(6):530-9.

Branco-de-Almeida LS, Kajiya M, Cardoso CR, Silva MJ, Ohta K, Rosalen PL, Franco GC, Han X, Taubman MA, Kawai T. Selective serotonin reuptake inhibitors attenuate the antigen presentation from dendritic cells to effector T lymphocytes. *FEMS Immunol. Med. Microbiol.* 2011 Aug;62(3):283-94.

Brandes LJ, Arron RJ, Bogdanovic RP, Tong J, Zaborniak CL, Hogg GR, Warrington RC, Fang W, LaBella FS. Stimulation of malignant growth in rodents by antidepressant drugs at clinically relevant doses. *Cancer Res.* 1992 Jul 1;52(13):3796-800.

Cloonan SM, Drozgowska A, Fayne D, Williams DC. The antidepressants maprotiline and fluoxetine have potent selective antiproliferative effects against Burkitt lymphoma independently of the norepinephrine and serotonin transporters. *Leuk Lymphoma.* 2010 Mar;51(3):523-39.

Cloonan SM, Williams DC. The antidepressants maprotiline and fluoxetine induce Type II autophagic cell death in drug-resistant Burkitt's lymphoma. *Int. J. Cancer.* 2011 Apr 1;128(7):1712-23.

Crowson AN, Magro CM. Antidepressant therapy. A possible cause of atypical cutaneous lymphoid hyperplasia. *Arch. Dermatol.* 1995 Aug;131(8):925-9.

Diamond M, Kelly JP, Connor TJ. Antidepressants suppress production of the Th1 cytokine interferon-gamma, independent of monoamine transporter blockade. *Eur. Neuropsychopharmacol.* 2006 Oct;16(7):481-90.

Edgar VA, Cremaschi GA, Sterin-Borda L, Genaro AM. Altered expression of autonomic neurotransmitter receptors and proliferative responses in lymphocytes from a chronic mild stress model of depression: effects of fluoxetine. *Brain Behav. Immun.* 2002 Aug;16(4):333-50.

Edgar VA, Genaro AM, Cremaschi G, Sterin-Borda L. Fluoxetine action on murine T-lymphocyte proliferation: participation of PKC activation and calcium mobilisation. *Cell Signal* 1998;10:721-6.

Edgar VA, Sterin-Borda L, Cremaschi GA, Genaro AM. Role of protein kinase C and cAMP in fluoxetine effects on human T-cell proliferation. *Eur. J. Pharmacol.* 1999;372:65-73.

Fazzino F, Montes C, Urbina M, Carreira I, Lima L. Serotonin transporter is differentially localized in subpopulations of lymphocytes of major depression patients. Effect of fluoxetine on proliferation. *J. Neuroimmunol.* 2008 May 30;196(1-2):173-80.

Fazzino F, Urbina M, Cedeño N, Lima L. Fluoxetine treatment to rats modifies serotonin transporter and cAMP in lymphocytes, CD4+ and CD8+ subpopulations and interleukins 2 and 4. *Int. Immunopharmacol.* 2009 Apr;9(4):463-7.

Fisch MJ, Loehrer PJ, Kristeller J, Passik S, Jung SH, Shen J, Arquette MA, Brames MJ, Einhorn LH; Hoosier Oncology Group. Fluoxetine versus placebo in advanced cancer outpatients: a double-blinded trial of the Hoosier Oncology Group. *J. Clin. Oncol.* 2003 May 15;21(10):1937-43.

Frank MG, Hendricks SE, Johnson DR, Wieseler JL, Burke WJ. Antidepressants augment natural killer cell activity: in vivo and in vitro. *Neuropsychobiology* 1999;39(1):18-24.

Freire-Garabal M, Nuñez MJ, Losada C, Pereiro D, Riveiro MP, González-Patiño E, Mayán JM, Rey-Mendez M. Effects of fluoxetine on the immunosuppressive response to stress in mice. *Life Sci.* 1997;60(26): PL403-13.

Freire-Garabal M, Núñez MJ, Pereiro D, Riveiro P, Losada C, Fernández-Rial JC, García-Iglesias E, Prizmic J, Mayán JM, Rey-Méndez M. Effects of fluoxetine on the development of lung metastases induced by operative stress in rats. *Life Sci.* 1998;63(2):PL31-8.

Freire-Garabal M, Núñez MJ, Riveiro P, Balboa J, López P, Zamorano BG, Rodrigo E, Rey-Méndez M. Effects of fluoxetine on the activity of phagocytosis in stressed mice. *Life Sci.* 2002 Nov 29;72(2):173-83.

Freire-Garabal M, Rey-Méndez M, García-Vallejo LA, Balboa J, Suárez JM, Rodrigo E, Brenlla J, Núñez MJ. Effects of nefazodone on the development of experimentally induced tumors in stressed rodents. *Psychopharmacology (Berl).* 2004 Nov;176(3-4):233-8.

Frick LR, Arcos ML, Rapanelli M, Zappia MP, Brocco M, Mongini C, Genaro AM, Cremaschi GA. Chronic restraint stress impairs T-cell immunity and promotes tumor progression in mice. *Stress.* 2009a;12(2):134-43.

Frick LR, Palumbo ML, Zappia MP, Brocco MA, Cremaschi GA, Genaro AM. Inhibitory effect of fluoxetine on lymphoma growth through the modulation of antitumor T-cell response by serotonin-dependent and independent mechanisms. *Biochem. Pharmacol.* 2008 May 1;75(9): 1817-26.

Frick LR, Rapanelli M, Arcos ML, Cremaschi GA, Genaro AM. Oral administration of fluoxetine alters the proliferation/apoptosis balance of lymphoma cells and up-regulates T cell immunity in tumor-bearing mice. *Eur. J. Pharmacol.* 2011 Jun 1;659(2-3):265-72.

Frick LR, Rapanelli M, Cremaschi GA, Genaro AM. Fluoxetine directly counteracts the adverse effects of chronic stress on T cell immunity by compensatory and specific mechanisms. *Brain Behav. Immun.* 2009b Jan;23(1):36-40.

Friedman GD, Udaltsova N, Chan J, Quesenberry CP Jr, Habel LA. Screening pharmaceuticals for possible carcinogenic effects: initial positive results for drugs not previously screened. *Cancer Causes Control.* 2009 Dec;20(10):1821-35.

Genaro AM, Edgar VA, Sterin-Borda L. Differential effects of fluoxetine on murine B-cell proliferation depending on the biochemical pathways triggered by distinct mitogens. *Biochem. Pharmacol.* 2000;60:1279-83.

Gordon J, Barnes NM. Lymphocytes transport serotonin and dopamine: agony or ecstasy? *Trends Immunol.* 2003 Aug;24(8):438-43.

Holland JC, Romano SJ, Heiligenstein JH, Tepner RG, Wilson MG. A controlled trial of fluoxetine and desipramine in depressed women with advanced cancer. *Psychooncology* 1998 Jul-Aug;7(4):291-300.

Kubera M, Grygier B, Arteta B, Urbańska K, Basta-Kaim A, Budziszewska B, Leśkiewicz M, Kołaczkowska E, Maes M, Szczepanik M, Majewska M, Lasoń W. Age-dependent stimulatory effect of desipramine and fluoxetine pretreatment on metastasis formation by B16F10 melanoma in male C57BL/6 mice. *Pharmacol. Rep.* 2009 Nov-Dec;61(6):1113-26.

Kubera M, Simbirtsev A, Mathison R, Maes M. Effects of repeated fluoxetine and citalopram administration on cytokine release in C57BL/6 mice. *Psychiatry Res.* 2000;96:255-66.

Lawlor DA, Jüni P, Ebrahim S, Egger M. Systematic review of the epidemiologic and trial evidence of an association between antidepressant medication and breast cancer. *J. Clin. Epidemiol.* 2003 Feb;56(2):155-63.

Lee CS, Kim YJ, Jang ER, Kim W, Myung SC. Fluoxetine induces apoptosis in ovarian carcinoma cell line OVCAR-3 through reactive oxygen species-dependent activation of nuclear factor-kappaB. *Basic Clin. Pharmacol. Toxicol.* 2010 Jun;106(6):446-53.

Lee KM, Kim YK. The role of IL-12 and TGF-beta1 in the pathophysiology of major depressive disorder. *Int. Immunopharmacol.* 2006 Aug;6(8): 1298-304.

Levkovitz Y, Gil-Ad I, Zeldich E, Dayag M, Weizman A. Differential induction of apoptosis by antidepressants in glioma and neuroblastoma cell lines: evidence for p-c-Jun, cytochrome c, and caspase-3 involvement. *J. Mol. Neurosci.* 2005;27(1):29-42.

Lima L, Urbina M. Serotonin transporter modulation in blood lymphocytes from patients with major depression. *Cell Mol. Neurobiol.* 2002 Dec;22 (5-6):797-804.

Loprinzi CL, Sloan JA, Perez EA, Quella SK, Stella PJ, Mailliard JA, Halyard MY, Pruthi S, Novotny PJ, Rummans TA. Phase III evaluation of fluoxetine for treatment of hot flashes. *J. Clin. Oncol.* 2002 Mar 15;20(6):1578-83.

Mariani L, Quattrini M, Atlante M, Galati M, Barbati A, Giannarelli D. Hot-flashes in breast cancer survivors: effectiveness of low-dosage fluoxetine. A pilot study. *J. Exp. Clin. Cancer Res.* 2005 Sep;24(3):373-8.

Miguel C, Albuquerque E. Drug interaction in psycho-oncology: antidepressants and antineoplastics. *Pharmacology.* 2011;88(5-6):333-9.

Navari RM, Brenner MC, Wilson MN. Treatment of depressive symptoms in patients with early stage breast cancer undergoing adjuvant therapy. *Breast Cancer Res. Treat.* 2008 Nov;112(1):197-201.

Núñez MJ, Balboa J, Rodrigo E, Brenlla J, González-Peteiro M, Freire-Garabal M. Effects of fluoxetine on cellular immune response in stressed mice. *Neurosci. Lett.* 2006 Apr 3;396(3):247-51.

Peer D, Dekel Y, Melikhov D, Margalit R. Fluoxetine inhibits multidrug resistance extrusion pumps and enhances responses to chemotherapy in syngeneic and in human xenograft mouse tumor models. *Cancer Res.* 2004 Oct 15;64(20):7562-9.

Pellegrino TC, Bayer BM. Modulation of immune cell function following fluoxetine administration in rats. *Pharmacol. Biochem. Behav.* 1998 Jan;59(1):151-7.

Pellegrino TC, Bayer BM. Role of central 5-HT(2) receptors in fluoxetine-induced decreases in T lymphocyte activity. Brain Behav Immun. 2002 Apr;16(2):87-103.

Pellegrino TC, Bayer BM. Specific serotonin reuptake inhibitor-induced decreases in lymphocyte activity require endogenous serotonin release. *Neuroimmunomodulation.* 2000;8(4):179-87.

Ploppa A, Ayers DM, Johannes T, Unertl KE, Durieux ME. The inhibition of human neutrophil phagocytosis and oxidative burst by tricyclic antidepressants. *Anesth. Analg.* 2008 Oct;107(4):1229-35.

Serafeim A, Holder MJ, Grafton G, Chamba A, Drayson MT, Luong QT, Bunce CM, Gregory CD, Barnes NM, Gordon J. Selective serotonin reuptake inhibitors directly signal for apoptosis in biopsy-like Burkitt lymphoma cells. *Blood.* 2003 Apr 15;101(8):3212-9.

Sheehan PF, Baker T, Tutton PJ, Barkla DH. Effects of histamine and 5-hydroxytryptamine on the growth rate of xenografted human bronchogenic carcinomas. *Clin. Exp. Pharmacol. Physiol.* 1996 Jun-Jul;23(6-7):465-71.

Spanová A, Kovárů H, Lisá V, Lukásová E, Rittich B. Estimation of apoptosis in C6 glioma cells treated with antidepressants. *Physiol. Res.* 1997;46(2):161-4.

Steingart AB, Cotterchio M. Do antidepressants cause, promote, or inhibit cancers? *J. Clin. Epidemiol.* 1995 Nov;48(11):1407-12.

Stepulak A, Rzeski W, Sifringer M, Brocke K, Gratopp A, Kupisz K, Turski L, Ikonomidou C. Fluoxetine inhibits the extracellular signal regulated kinase pathway and suppresses growth of cancer cells. *Cancer Biol. Ther.* 2008 Oct;7(10):1685-93.

Strümper D, Durieux ME, Hollmann MW, Tröster B, den Bakker CG, Marcus MA. Effects of antidepressants on function and viability of human neutrophils. *Anesthesiology.* 2003 Jun;98(6):1356-62.

Toscano MA, Bianco GA, Ilarregui JM, Croci DO, Correale J, Hernandez JD, Zwirner NW, Poirier F, Riley EM, Baum LG, Rabinovich GA. Differential glycosylation of TH1, TH2 and TH-17 effector cells selectively regulates susceptibility to cell death. *Nat. Immunol.* 2007 Aug;8(8):825-34.

Tutton PJ, Barkla DH. Influence of inhibitors of serotonin uptake on intestinal epithelium and colorectal carcinomas. *Br. J. Cancer.* 1982 Aug;46(2): 260-5.

Volpe DA, Ellison CD, Parchment RE, Grieshaber CK, Faustino PJ. Effects of amitriptyline and fluoxetine upon the in vitro proliferation of tumor cell lines. *J. Exp. Ther. Oncol.* 2003 Jul-Aug;3(4):169-84.

Wallace WA, Balsitis M, Harrison BJ. Male breast neoplasia in association with selective serotonin re-uptake inhibitor therapy: a report of three cases. *Eur. J. Surg. Oncol.* 2001 Jun;27(4):429-31.

In: Antidepressants
Editors: L. J. Mígne and J. W. Post

ISBN: 978-1--62081-555-7
© 2012 Nova Science Publishers, Inc.

Chapter 5

USE OF ANTIDEPRESSANTS IN OLDER PEOPLE WITH MENTAL ILLNESS: A SYSTEMATIC STUDY OF TOLERABILITY AND USE IN DIFFERENT DIAGNOSTIC GROUPS

Stephen Curran[1], Debbie Turner[2], Shabir Musa[3], Andrew Byrne[2], and John Wattis[4]*

[1]Ageing and Mental Health Research Group, School of Human and Health Sciences, University of Huddersfield, and South West Yorkshire Mental Health NHS Trust, Wakefield, UK
[2]Calder Unit, South West Yorkshire Mental Health NHS Trust, Wakefield, UK
[3]Chantry Unit, South West Yorkshire Mental Health NHS Trust, Wakefield, UK
[4]Ageing and Mental Health Research Unit, School of Human and Health Sciences, University of Huddersfield, and South West Yorkshire Mental Health NHS Trust, St Luke's Hospital, Huddersfield, UK

---

* Address for correspondence: Professor Stephen Curran; Ageing and Mental Health Research Group, HW3-02; Harold Wilson Building; School of Human and Health Sciences; University of Huddersfield, HD1 3DH; Huddersfield; UK; Tel: 01484 472443; Fax: 01484 473 760; Email: s.curran@hud.ac.uk

ABSTRACT

Aims: The objective of the study was to provide observational clinical data on psychotropic drugs used in older people with mental illness.

Method: This was an observational, single-centre, one-week prevalence study of psychiatric symptoms, disorders and psychotropic/ antidepressant drug use in older people with mental illness cared for by the South West people Yorkshire Mental Health NHS Trust (Wakefield Locality), UK. The clinical assessment included completion of the Psychosis Evaluation Tool for Common use by Caregivers.

Results: A total of 593/660 older patients with mental illness (mean±SD age, 76±8.1 years) were assessed). 44.5% had dementia (excluding vascular dementia) and 33.7% had a mood disorder. Of the total, 20.4% did not receive CNS active medication and 46.2% of patients were prescribed an antidepressant. Antidepressants were commonly prescribed where the primary diagnosis was not depression including vascular dementia (31%), dementia (26.1%), schizophrenia and related disorders (26.2%) and anxiety disorders (51.5%). SSRIs were the most commonly prescribed drugs (63.2%) followed by TCAs (22.4%), venlafaxine (9%), mirtazapine (3.2%), reboxetine (1.8%) and phenelzine (0.36%). The single most commonly prescribed drug was paroxetine (n=77) which accounted for 27.7% of all prescriptions. Medications were well tolerated but some patients prescribed a TCA received relatively small doses. Patients with non-vascular dementia received a significantly lower dose of paroxetine compared with other diagnostic groups (F=3.14, p<0.02) though this was still within the recommended/therapeutic range.

Conclusions: Antidepressants are commonly used in older people with mental illness including dementia, schizophrenia and anxiety disorders as well as for patients with a primary diagnosis of depression. Antidepressants are generally well tolerated and patients were broadly satisfied with their medication. The evidence for the use of low dose TCAs in older people remains controversial and further work is needed in this area.

Declaration of interest: None

Keywords: psychotropics, antidepressants, older people, mental illness

Depression in older people is similar to major depression at other times of life. However ageing and other factors may alter the presentation of depression in later life. In particular older people are less likely to complain of sadness compared with younger patients, they are more likely to complain of physical symptoms (NIH, 1992), memory complaints and anxiety symptoms (Baldwin et al., 2002).

In addition, depression in patients with dementia is a common cause of behavioural disturbance (Dwyer and Byrne, 2000). Depression is one of the leading causes of disability, leads to a greater risk of hospitalisation as well as prolonging hospitalisation and is the single most important predictor of suicide. It also reduces compliance with medical treatments, reduces the patient's quality of life and is an independent predictor of mortality (Baldwin et al., 2002).

Depression in older people is two to three times more prevalent than dementia (Katona, 1994) and is the most common mental health problem amongst older adults. In community samples the prevalence of mild depression has been estimated to be 11% (Alexopoulous, 1992) rising to 22-33% in residential and nursing homes (Ames et al., 1988) and 45% in hospitalised elderly patients with physical illness (Koenig et al., 1988). There is also some evidence of increased prevalence in the very old (Stek et al., 2006).

The aetiology of depression in older people is complex. Genetic susceptibility is less important compared with younger patients. Female gender, a previous history of depression and loss of spouse increases susceptibility. Reductions in levels of noradrenaline and serotonin, decreases in brain weight and the greater prevalence of deep white matter and subcortical grey matter lesions all play a part. Hypertension, vascular risk factors, impaired function, being chronically ill and being a carer are also important risk factors as are life events such as bereavement, separation, acute physical illness and moving into residential care.

A number of drugs can also cause or aggravate depression including beta-blockers, methyldopa, calcium channel blockers, digoxin and steroids (NIH, 1992; Jonas and Mussolino, 2000; Ariyo et al., 2000; Penninx et al., 2000; Baldwin et al., 2002). For these reasons, antidepressants are usually only part of the solution for the treatment of depression in older people.

In a recent Canadian study (Beck et al., 2005) the prevalence of psychotropic drug use in the general population was 7.2% and selective serotonin reuptake inhibitors and venlafaxine accounted for 25.2% of all psychotropic drug usage. Although there is now a reasonably good body of evidence for the efficacy of antidepressants in older people (Wilson et al., 2001; Oslin et al., 2003; Guaiang et al., 2004; Sheikh et al., 2004; Nelson, 2005) very little information has been published on the use of antidepressants in this age group.

The aim of the present study was to provide a better understanding of psychotropic drug use and particularly antidepressant use in older people with mental illness as well as exploring tolerability and prescribing issues in different diagnostic groups.

METHOD

Study Design

This was an observational, single-centre, one week prevalence study of psychiatric symptoms, disorders and psychotropic drug use carried out in the Wakefield Locality, South West Yorkshire Mental Health NHS Trust, UK over 12 months in 2003/2004. The service consisted of two acute wards, one day-hospital, outpatient clinics for three consultant teams, three Community Units for the Elderly, and two Community Mental Health Teams. The study was approved by the Wakefield Research Ethics Committee.

Patient Selection

All consenting patients under the care of psychiatric services for older people in the Wakefield Locality (total population over 65 years approximately 55,000) were included in the study. Patients identified from Trust records were contacted by a Research Nurse to ask if they would like to take part in the study.

All patients and caregivers received an information sheet before taking part in the study and gave written consent.

Assessments

The Research Nurse undertook a detailed clinical assessment, which included demographic details, clinical information, diagnosis and treatment response (classified as first episode, stable-dissatisfied, stable-satisfied, treatment resistant, and uncontrolled), medication, symptoms and side-effects. These were part of a computer-based package, the Psychosis Evaluation Tool for Common use by Caregivers (PECC), developed from the work of Lindstrom et al. (1997).

The PECC was specifically designed to be used by a wide variety of health care workers including nurses. The reliability and validity has been described in both younger and older people (de Hert et al., 1999). Prior to undertaking the study the Research Nurse attended a three-day training course organised by the PECC development team in Belgium.

The assessment also included an interview with the caregiver, discussions with medical and nursing staff and a review of medical notes including GP records. This specifically included a review of patients' current physical health and laboratory and other investigations.

Patients were assessed in a variety of settings including the two acute wards, OP clinics, the three Community Units for the Elderly and in their own homes. The assessment took approximately one hour to complete and after the assessment a copy was made available to the appropriate clinical team. Diagnosis was based on DSM-IVR criteria (APA, 1994). Some patients attended several parts of the service e.g. day hospital and OP clinic but they were only included once.

Symptoms and side-effects were based on the previous seven days and a standardised protocol was used for *defining* and *scoring* individual symptoms and side-effects.

Symptoms were recorded on a seven-point scale (1=absent, 7=extreme burden, all areas of functioning are disturbed, supervision necessary) and included positive (e.g. delusions and hallucinations) and negative symptoms (e.g. motor retardation, blunted affect, poor rapport and passive social withdrawal) as well as depressive, cognitive and excitatory symptoms. Side-effects were measured on a four-point scale (1=absent; 4=severe, obvious influence on functioning, intervention necessary) and included extrapyramidal side-effects (EPS), anticholinergic, hormonal, dizziness, daytime somnolence, drowsiness, sexual dysfunction, insomnia, weight gain and orthostatic hypotension.

Statistical Analysis

Statistical analyses were carried out using SAS/STAT software (version 8.12). Comparisons of continuous variable used ANOVA, and pair-wise comparisons (Chi squared test - χ^2, Cochran-Mantel-Haenzel test) for categorical variables were performed with adjustment for multiple comparisons employing the Tukey-Kramer's method.

RESULTS

Patient Characteristics

Of a total of 660 older patients, 593 (89.8%) patients took part in the study. 293 patients (approximately 50%) had a diagnosis of dementia with 4.9% of the total population having vascular dementia (VaD). Of the remaining patients 200 (33.7%) had an affective disorder and 65 (11%) schizophrenia or a related disorder. In addition, the majority of patients had had their mental illness for a relatively short period (table 1).

Age of the patients ranged from 44 to 97 years, the mean age±SD was 76±8.1years, and 44% were aged 71 to 80 years. There was a statistical difference in the age of the patients between the diagnostic groups (F=8.37, p<0.001). More specifically, patients with VaD and non vascular dementia were older than patients with affective disorders (p=0.035, p<0.001, respectively) and were older than those with schizophrenia and related disorders (p<0.0005).

Sixty-nine percent (n=409) of patients were female and there were more females (≥67%) in each diagnostic category (χ^2, p=0.001), with the exception of VaD dementia (males n=19, 65.5%; females n=10, 34.5%).

Table 1. Frequency distribution of main diagnoses and time in years since the main diagnosis was made

Diagnosis	Main diagnosis n (%) patients	Time in years since main diagnosis Mean ±SD years (range)
Vascular dementia	29 (4.9)	0.4±0.8 (0-4.0)
Non vascular dementia	264 (44.5)	0.5±1.2 (0-8.9)
Affective disorders	200 (33.7)	0.4±0.9 (0-7.3)
Schizophrenia, schizotypal and delusional disorders	65 (11.0)	1.7±5.0 (0-28.0)
Anxiety disorders	33 (5.6)	0.3±0.3 (0-0.9)
Unknown	2 (0.3)	1.2±1.3 (0.3-2.1)
Total	593 (100)	0.6±2.0 (0-28)

There were no differences in the level of education, occupational status or marital status between the diagnostic groups. Treatment response was rated as "stable-satisfied" for the majority of patients (n=537, 90.6%) with 7 patients (1.2%) rated as "stable-dissatisfied."

Only 2 patients (0.3%) were rated at "treatment resistant." The time in years since patients were first diagnosed with their principal mental disorder ranged from 0 to 28 years. This was numerically greater for patients with schizophrenia and related disorders but there were no statistically significant differences between the diagnostic groups (p=0.97 - table 1).

Psychoactive Drugs

Of the 593 patients, 121 (20.4%) did not receive a psychoactive drug. A total of 304 (51.3%) patients were taking an antipsychotic, 274 (46.2%) an antidepressant, 130 (21.9%) an hypnotic, 42 (7.1%) an anxiolytic, 29 (4.7%) an anticonvulsant and 29 (4.9%) anticholinergic drugs.

Intake of Antidepressants

In total 46.2% of patients were prescribed an antidepressant and these were more likely to be prescribed to patients with depression (81%) compared with other diagnoses (VaD 31%, dementia 26.1%, schizophrenia and related disorders 26.2% and anxiety disorders 51.5%) (χ^2=155.5, p<0.001). SSRIs were the most commonly prescribed drugs (63.2%) followed by TCAs (22.4%), venlafaxine (9%), mirtazapine (3.2%), reboxetine (1.8%) and phenelzine (0.36%).

The single most commonly prescribed drug was paroxetine (n=77) and this accounted for 27.7% of all prescriptions. All antidepressants were prescribed in therapeutic doses although some patients prescribed a TCA received subtherapeutic doses.

The mean daily doses for the most commonly prescribed TCAs were amitriptyline (mean 62.8 mg, range 50-150 mg), doxepin (mean 100 mg, range 50-150 mg), imipramine (mean 66.7 mg, range 25-150 mg and lofepramine (mean 131.3 mg, range 140-210 mg).

In addition use of sertraline (F=1.34, p<0.27) and fluoxetine (F=0.71, p<0.55) did not differ significantly between the diagnostic groups. However, patients with dementia received a significantly lower dose of paroxetine compared with other diagnostic groups (F=3.14, p<0.02) though this was still within the recommended/therapeutic range.

Evaluation of Symptoms

There were significant differences between the different diagnosis groups for the mean scores of cognitive (F=56.7, p<0.001), depressive (F=44.4, p<0.001), negative (F=8.5, p<0.001), and positive (F=27.9, p<0.001) symptoms (table 2). Not unexpectedly, patients with dementia had more problems with cognitive function, those with affective disorders had greater depressive symptoms, and negative and positive symptoms were greatest in patients with schizophrenia and related disorders.

Excitatory symptoms (e.g. hyperactivity, agitation, poor impulse control and hostility) were not significantly different between the diagnostic groups (F=2.1, p= 0.08) (table 2).

Table 2. Symptom scores (1=absent, 7=extreme burden, all areas of functioning are disturbed, supervision necessary) Mean score ±SD

Diagnosis	Cognitive Depressive Excitatory Negative Positive
Vascular dementia (n=29)	1.277 1.121 1.078 1.129 1.043 ±0.208 ±0.207 ±0.178 ±0.456 ±0.150
Non vascular dementia (n=264)	1.354 1.150 1.054 1.046 1.106 ±0.200 ±0.251 ±0.160 ±0.189 ±0.208
Affective disorders (n=200)	1.077 1.649 1.032 1.181 1.078 ±0.167 ±0.552 ±0.183 ±0.399 ±0.194
Schizophrenia, schizotypal and delusional disorders (n=65)	1.173 1.349 1.108 1.254 1.450 ±0.353 ±0.526 ±0.334 ±0.450 ±0.559
Anxiety disorders (n=33)	1.053 1.583 1.039 1.045 1.061 ±0.104 ±0.499 ±0.129 ±0.159 ±0.166
Total (n=593)	1.219 1.363 1.052 1.118 1.129 ±0.245 ±0.480 ±0.194 ±0.329 ±0.285

Evaluation of Side-Effects

Medication was generally well tolerated but anticholinergic side-effects (range 1-3) and drowsiness (1-2.4) were significantly higher in patients with an affective disorder compared with other diagnoses (F=2.9, p=0.02 and F=7.8, p<0.001 respectively).

DISCUSSION

The principal objective of this study was to obtain a better understanding of the use and tolerability of psychotropic drugs in older people and this paper makes particular reference to antidepressants. The study was undertaken just before the CSM guidance was issued on venlafaxine (CSM, 2004). Antidepressants drugs are commonly used in older people with mental illness including dementia, schizophrenia and related disorders and anxiety disorders as well as for depression.

It is interesting that there were no differences in the level of education, occupational status or marital status between the diagnostic groups. The time in years since patients were first diagnosed with their main mental disorder was relatively short and ranged from 0 to 28 years. It is likely that since most patients developed their illness later in life this did not have a significant impact on their education and life choices such as occupation and marriage. In addition over 90% of patients reported feeling "satisfied" with their treatment. Seven percent reported feeling "dissatisfied" and 2% were classified as treatment resistant. The definition of treatment resistant depression (TRD) was not clearly defined in this study. Overall this is probably an underestimate of the true prevalence of TRD. However, the main focus of this study was drug use and tolerability rather than efficacy.

This study confirms that antidepressants are commonly prescribed to older people with mental illness. 46.2% of patients were prescribed an antidepressant and whilst the largest proportion was for patients with depression, 26.1% of patients with dementia, 26.2% with schizophrenia and related disorders and 51.5% of patients with an anxiety disorder received an antidepressant. A wide range of antidepressants were prescribed and of those prescribed an antidepressant six patients (2.2%) were prescribed two. The most commonly prescribed antidepressant was paroxetine which was prescribed at lower doses in older patients with dementia compared with other diagnoses. In addition, doses of TCAs tended to be lower compared with other antidepressants. However, in a relatively recent Cochrane review Furukawa et al. (2004) concluded that low dose TCAs can be justified though the debate on this issue has not concluded. Antidepressants were generally well tolerated but patients with depression reported significantly more drowsiness and anticholinergic side-effects compared with other diagnostic groups. Clinicians need clear advice on the use of antidepressant in older people. This advice should be based on good quality efficacy, tolerability and safety data from randomised-controlled studies and more research is needed in this area.

ACKNOWLEDGMENTS

This was an Investigator Initiated Project funded by an unconditional educational grant from Janssen-Cilag (UK).

REFERENCES

Alexopoulous G S. (1992) Geriatric depression reaches maturity. *International Journal of Geriatric Psychiatry,* 1992; 7:305-306.

American Psychiatric Association (1994) *Diagnostic and Statistical Manual of Mental Disorders,* Third Edition (Revised), Washington, D.C.

Ames D, Ashby D, Mann AH, Graham N. (1988) Psychiatric illness in elderly residents of part 3 homes in one London borough: prognosis and review. *Age and Ageing,* 1988; 17(4):249-256.

Ariyo AA, haan M, Tangen CM et al. (2000) Depressive symptoms and risks of coronary heart disease and mortality in elderly Americans. *Circulation,* 102, 1773-1779.

Baldwin RC, Chiu, E, Katona, C, Grahaam, N. (2002) *Guidelines on Depression in Older People: practising the evidence.* Martin Dunitz, London 2002.

Beck CA, Williams JV, Wang JL et al. (2005) Psychotropic medication use in Canada. *Canadian Journal of Psychiatry,* 50(10), 605-613.

Committee on Safety of Medicines (2004) *Safety of Selective Serotonin Reuptake Inhibitor Antidepressants.* www.mhra.gov.uk.

de Hert M, Bussels J, Lindstrom E, Abrahams F, Fransens C and Peuskens J. 1999. PECC Psychosis Evaluation Tool for Common use by Caregivers. Drukkerji EPO: Berchem. Dwyer M and Byrne GJ (2000) Disruptive vocalisation and depression in older nursing home residents. *International Psychogeriatrics,* 12, 463-471.

Furukawa T, McGuire H and Barbui C (2004) Low dosage tricyclic antidepressants for depression. *Cochrane Review.* 3, 2004.

Guaiana G, Barbui C and Hotopf M. (2004) Amitriptyline versus other types of pharmacotherapy for depression. *Cochrane Review.* 3, 2004.

Jonas BS and Mussolino ME (2000) Symptoms of depression as a prospective risk factor for stroke. Psychosomatic Medicine, 62, 463-471.

Katona CLE. (1994) The Epidemiology of depression in old age. *Depression in old age.* Chichester: John Wiley and son, 1994: 29-42.

Koenig H G, Meador K G, Cohen H J , Blazer D. (1988) Depression in elderly hospitalised patients with medical illness. *Archives of Internal Medicine,* 1988; 148: 1929-1936.

Lindstrom E, Ekselius l, Jedenius E, Almqvist A and Wieselgren IM. 1997. A checklist for assessment of treatment in schizophrenia syndromes; interscale validity and interrater reliability. *Primary Care Psychiatry.* 3: 183-187.

National Institute for Health (1992) NIH Consensus Panel. Diagnosis and treatment of depression in late life. *Journal of the American Medical Association,* 268, 1018-1024.

Nelson JC, Wohlreich MM, Mallinckrodt CH et al. (2005) Duloxetine for the treatment of major depressive disorder in older people. *American Journal of Geriatric Psychiatry,* 13(3), 227-235.

Oslin DW, Have TRT, Streim JE et al. (2003) Probing the safety of medications in the frail elderly; evidence from a randomised clinical trial of sertraline and venlafaxine in depressed nursing home residents. *Journal of Clinical Psychiatry,* 2003; 64(8):875-882.

Penninx BW, Deeg DJ, van Eijk JT et al. (2000) Changes in depression and physical decline in older adults; a londitudinal perspective. *Journal of Affective Disorders,* 61, 1-12.

Sheikh JI, Cassidy EL, Doraiswamy PM et al. (2004) Efficacy, safety and tolerability of sertraline in patients with late-life depression. *Journal of the American Geriatrics Society,* 2004; 52(1): 86-92.

Steck ML, Vinkers DJ, Gussekloo J et al. (2006) Natural history of depression in the oldest old. *British Journal of Psychiatry,* 188, 65-69.

Wilson K, Mottram P, Sivanranthan A, Nightingale A. (2001) Antidepressant versus placebo for depressed elderly (Cochrane Review). In: *The Cochrane Library,* 2001; Issue 2. Oxford: Update Software.

In: Antidepressants   ISBN: 978-1--62081-555-7
Editors: L. J. Mígne and J. W. Post   © 2012 Nova Science Publishers, Inc.

Chapter 6

TREATMENT OF COMORBID DEPRESSION AND ALCOHOL ABUSE/DEPENDENCE WITH ANTIDEPRESSANT MEDICATIONS

Thomas Paparrigopoulos, *Eleftherios Mellos,* *and Ioannis Liappas*

Athens University Medical School,
1st Department of Psychiatry, Eginition Hospital, Athens, Greece

INTRODUCTION

Alcohol use disorders are often accompanied by symptoms of other major psychiatric syndromes which may precede, follow, or be concurrent but independent of alcohol misuse. Epidemiological and clinical studies provide evidence that at least two-thirds of alcohol abusing individuals present with clinically significant symptoms of anxiety, sadness, mania-like conditions, other substance use disorders and antisocial behaviours [1, 2, 3, 4]. Affective disorders, including major depression, dysthymia or bipolar disorder, have been shown to be among the most frequent psychiatric disorders that co-occur with alcohol dependence [3, 5, 6, 7]. It is reported that in community samples there is a 2- to 4-fold greater lifetime risk for developing one disorder when

* Corresponding author: Thomas Paparrigopoulos, Athens University Medical School, 1st Department of Psychiatry, Eginition Hospital, Vas. Sofias 74, Athens 115 28, Greece, Tel./ Fax: +210 7289324. E-mail: tpaparrig@med.uoa.gr.

the other disorder is present and that this risk is even higher in treatment settings [8]. The co-occurrence of affective and alcohol disorders aggravates the clinical course, treatment outcome, and prognosis for each one of them. Individuals with both disorders have significantly increased rates of alcohol relapse, more severe symptoms, increased suicide risk, poorer treatment compliance and response, severe social and occupational impairment and disability, and consequently higher health services costs [9, 10, 11, 12, 13]. In this context, a growing literature related to the treatment of comorbid depression and alcohol dependence has developed during the last decade, which suggests that antidepressants could be of help in the management of depressed alcoholics.

PREVALENCE OF COMORBID DEPRESSION AND ALCOHOL DEPENDENCE

Although a large variability attributed to methodological or diagnostic issues exists, findings from both clinical and epidemiological surveys have clearly demonstrated the extent of comorbidity between alcohol abuse/dependence and depressive disorders. Results from clinical studies may not be applicable to the general population, as clinical studies are often biased toward the more severely affected population. Therefore, estimates of comorbidity based on general population studies are considered to be more reliable [14].

The Epidemiological Catchment Area Survey (ECA) [15] was the first large-scale epidemiological study designed to collect information on the prevalence of mental disorders in the U.S. Approximately 20000 adults were assessed. Among respondents with a lifetime diagnosis of any alcohol use disorder, 37% had at least another comorbid mental disorder and conversely 22% with any lifetime mental disorder had a lifetime history of a concomitant alcohol use disorder. In specialist treatment settings, individuals with an alcohol use disorder were nearly four times as likely to have a comorbid mental disorder compared to individuals not in treatment. Regarding depression in particular, 16.5% of the individuals with lifetime major depression had an alcohol use disorder, and the prevalence of lifetime major depression in alcohol dependent individuals was 5% and 19% for men and women respectively.

These findings have been replicated several times, although the rate of comorbidity between the two conditions may vary considerably among different studies depending on methodology. Thus, data from the Collaborative Study on the Genetics of Alcoholism indicated that lifetime prevalence of major depressive disorder among treatment-seeking alcoholics was 42.2%, but that lifetime rate for independent major depression among alcoholics dropped to 15.2%, (a percentage close to that referred for the general population) with the remaining 26.4% reporting substance-induced major depression [16]. In the National Comorbidity Survey (NCS) [2] the estimate for alcohol dependence was 14.1% and for drug dependence 7.5%. Lifetime odds of alcohol dependence were significantly elevated for both men (2.95) and women (4.05) with major depression compared to non-depressed individuals, and a twofold increase of depression among subjects with alcohol dependence. In another large US survey, the National Longitudinal Alcohol Epidemiologic Survey (NLAES), 32.5% of the individuals with major depression met criteria for a lifetime diagnosis of alcohol dependence vs. 11.2% of those who did not meet criteria for major depression (3). Finally, data from the National Epidemiologic Survey on Alcohol and Related Conditions (NESARC), a recent large US survey covering the comorbidity of DSM-IV substance use disorders and mood / anxiety disorders, have shown significant 12-month and lifetime associations between alcohol use disorders and any mood disorder (odds ratio >2.2 and 2.4, respectively). Of clinical importance is the finding that 40.7% of the respondents with a current alcohol use disorder who sought treatment during the same period had at least one independent mood disorder [17].

Other North American and Australian studies have also recorded similarly high comorbidity rates. For instance the Ontario Health Survey reported that 28.1% of alcoholics vs. 8.6% of non-alcoholics had a lifetime major depressive episode [18]. Furthermore, according to the Canadian National Population Health Survey, being young (12-24 years), single and of low family income are potential risk factors for the co-occurrence of major depression and alcohol abuse [14]. Likewise, data from the US National Longitudinal Alcohol Epidemiologic Survey suggest that, compared with subjects with major depression, those with comorbid alcohol abuse/ dependence are younger, more likely to be male and less likely to be black. [19]. Finally, findings from the cross-sectional Australian National Survey of Mental Health and Well Being indicate that individuals with an alcohol use disorder are 10 times more likely to have another drug use disorder, 4 times more likely to have an affective disorder and 3 times more likely to have an anxiety disorder; also, respondents with comorbid disorders were more likely to be female, younger, employed and to have completed less years of secondary schooling [20].

PRIMARY VERSUS ALCOHOL-INDUCED DEPRESSION: CLINICAL ISSUES

A number of studies have supported that the depressive symptomatology observed among alcoholics represents a heterogeneous group of syndromes with different aetiology, clinical characteristics, prognoses and treatment needs [16, 21]. According to the Diagnostic and Statistical Manual of Mental Disorders, Fourth Edition (DSM-IV), a depressive disorder can be characterized either as primary or secondary or substance-induced [22]. A depressive episode is primary (or independent) if depressive symptoms precede the onset of alcohol use or persists for more than 4 weeks after the cessation of alcohol use. In contrast, secondary depressive episodes (or alcohol-induced) are defined as those occurring only during periods of alcohol abuse due to the pharmacological effects of heavy alcohol consumption, showing a marked and fairly rapid improvement following abstinence. Although in most cases secondary depression will remit with abstinence from alcohol, its persistence is still a possibility [23]. For instance, according to Ramsey's study, more than a quarter of depressive episodes originally diagnosed as secondary were reclassified as primary during the first year follow-up, obviously because of the prolongation of symptoms during abstinence. In their study, the authors found that clinical predictors of a substance-induced episode reclassification as independent were a history of past independent depression and a lower severity of alcohol dependence [24].

Several clinical studies, mainly of the 80's and 90's, support the view that 40% to 60% of mood disorders encountered in alcoholics represent temporary depressive episodes related to the repeated heavy alcohol intoxication (alcohol-induced depression) [1, 25, 26, 27].

Results from a 1997 report from the Collaborative Study on the Genetics of Alcoholism (phase II) corroborate a high rate of substance-induced major depressive episode, with these disorders explaining about half of the lifetime depressive episodes [25].

However, more recent epidemiological studies suggest that most mood disorders are independent of substance use instead. Data from NESARC, the largest comorbidity study based on the DSM-IV definitions of independent and alcohol-induced disorders, indicate that less than 1% of the general population had a substance-induced depressive episode during the last 12 months. Moreover, 40.7% of the individuals with a current alcohol use disorder who sought treatment during that period had at least another independent mood disorder [17]. Different results may reflect differences between the prevalence of alcohol use in general population and special population studies, the time frame of the studies (lifetime vs. one-year, cross-sectional), the type of interview used for the assessment, and apparently the changing pattern of alcohol use and consequently of concomitant psycho-pathology over the years [25]. Some cues can be useful in differentiating the two conditions. Thus, alcohol dependent individuals with independent major depression are more likely than those with substance-induced depression to: a) have a family history of independent depressive episodes, b) consume less alcohol, c) have a mild history of drug abuse, d) have received less treatment for alcohol abuse, e) have attempted suicide, f) have a younger age at onset of depression and longer depressive episodes, and g) have a different demo-graphic profile, i.e., are more often married white women [16, 25, 28, 29]. Distinguishing between independent and substance-induced psychopatho-logical conditions is often a difficult and complicated task [6, 8, 26]. Symptoms of intoxication or withdrawal associated with alcohol abuse can closely resemble independent psychiatric syndromes [8, 23, 26]. Schuckit suggests four key steps in attempting to differentiate independent vs. substance-induced psychopathology. The first step is to determine whether the patient fits actual criteria for an additional psychiatric disorder or his/her symptoms are temporary psychiatric manifestations. The second step is to clarify the approximate age at onset of each disorder and to establish the time course of each major disorder. The third step is to observe the course of mood symptoms during periods of abstinence, and last, the individual should be monitored for an extended period of time in order to know better the course of the psychiatric symptomatology [30].

RELATIONSHIP BETWEEN DEPRESSION AND ALCOHOL DEPENDENCE

Given the frequent co-occurrence of alcohol use disorders and major depression, understanding the nature of their relationship is important. Several hypotheses have been proposed in order to explain this type of comorbidity. In general, they fit in three categories: a) one condition may foster the other, b) the two conditions may be comorbid because they share common risk factors, and c) the two conditions may be correlated because they are manifestations of a common underlying syndrome or vulnerability [1, 8, 16, 31, 32, 33].

The explanation most frequently advanced for the co-occurrence of alcohol abuse and affective disorders is the phenotypic causation viewpoint, which suggests that each condition increases the risk for the development of the other [8, 33, 34]. According to this group of hypotheses, alcohol use represents an attempt to abate depressive symptoms (self-medication hypothesis) and conversely that the toxic and depressogenic effects of ethanol or the negative social and interpersonal consequences caused by alcohol abuse enhances the risk for developing depression. An alternative hypothesis is that comorbidity arises through common underlying factors, which may be either genetic or social and environmental [35, 36]. This aetiological relationship is illustrated by the findings of Tambs et al. study, which demonstrated that in the male population the correlation between substance abuse and depression can be wholly explained by shared genetic factors, whereas in the female population this correlation could be explained by the interaction between family, environmental and genetic factors [37]. Common genetic pre-disposition is further corroborated by the Collaborative Study on the Genetics of Alcoholism (COGA). In this large scale family study, designed to identify genes related to the risk for alcoholism and alcohol-related traits, including depressive symptomatology, the phenotype characterized by co-occurring alcoholism and depression showed evidence of linkage to a region on chromosome 2 [38]. Also, the broad alcoholism or depression phenotype showed evidence of linkage to the same region of chromosome 1 that was linked to alcoholism alone. These findings indicate that genes within this chromosomal region may predispose some individuals to alcoholism and others to depression [39].

GENERAL CONSIDERATIONS ON THE MANAGEMENT OF COMORBID DEPRESSION AND ALCOHOL DEPENDENCE

Treating individuals with comorbid depressive and alcohol disorders is a challenging and sometimes complex therapeutic process. Formerly, it was common practice to avoid prescribing antidepressant medications and efforts focused mainly on abstinence from alcohol [23, 26]. This viewpoint was held for various reasons, such as the widespread conviction in the transient nature of depressive symptoms, the stigma associated with giving medications to substance dependent individuals and the poor results reported by early treatment studies that evaluated antidepressants in depressed alcoholics [23, 40, 41]. However, during the last decade better controlled trials provided evidence of the efficacy of antidepressants for the management of depression among alcohol abusing or dependent individuals [23].

Clarifying the exact nature of depressive symptoms in alcoholics is important for determining the course of the illness and the optimal therapeutic approach [42]. Thus, in alcoholics with primary depression, psychopathology usually persists even after treating alcohol dependence. In such cases, untreated depression, following abstinence from alcohol, may be a risk factor for relapse to drinking as well as for suicidal attempts [23, 42]. Consequently, the use of antidepressants seems warranted. On the other hand, whenever the depressive symptomatology is related to alcohol use, it is debatable whether administration of antidepressants would have any therapeutic impact beyond what abstinence would achieve [23, 43]. This results from the well documented observation of a rapid reduction of depressive and anxiety symptoms following detoxification over a 2 to 4-week period of abstinence from alcohol [44, 45, 46]. Our own data collected from a group of alcoholics who were treated for alcohol abuse/dependence on an inpatient basis corroborate this finding [47]. In our sample, alcohol abusing patients evidenced a highly significant reduction on the Hamilton depression and anxiety scale scores and a considerable amelioration of overall functioning over the 4-5 weeks of detoxification. As far as symptoms of depression concern, a significant negative correlation was observed between the end score on the Hamilton depression scale and the age at onset of alcoholism, which is an indication that a better outcome was achieved in the case of subjects with a later onset of alcoholism [47]. However, of particular clinical interest is the fact that a significant percentage of depressive episodes classified as alcohol-induced do not remit after abstinence from alcohol, which increases the risk for relapse to drinking [24]. Thus, even in alcoholics with secondary depression antidepressant treatment may be indicated.

As a rule, management of alcohol dependence with comorbid depression includes alcohol detoxification and a combination of pharmacological and psychosocial approaches. This strategy aims at either achieving and maintaining abstinence or maximizing harm reduction, in parallel with the reduction of depressive symptoms. To this end, integration of pertinent services is crucial to achieve optimal therapeutic efficacy [6]. In particular, the psychotherapeutic/psychosocial management should be tailored to the individuals' needs and contain elements combined from the treatment of addictions and affective disorders [6]. Typically it includes counseling, dynamically oriented therapies, cognitive-behavioral therapies and interventions designed to enhance motivation to sobriety [11]. Cognitive-behavioral therapies are among the most effective psychosocial treatments for affective disorders and their efficacy has also been demonstrated in the treatment of alcohol dependence [48, 49]. Specific psychotherapeutic strategies of the cognitive-behavioral type have been developed for subjects with co-occurring disorders [50]. Brown found that cognitive-behavioral therapy was effective not only in improving depression, but in decreasing the frequency of drinking in alcoholics with severe symptoms of depression [50]. Another approach, motivational interviewing, has been also shown to be an effective therapeutic intervention in the cases of substance abuse with comorbid affective symptoms [6, 51]. Project MATCH demonstrated that in a 12-week outpatient trial of a large sample of alcoholics, cognitive-behavioral therapy or 12-step facilitation achieved better results compared to the motivational enhancement therapeutic approach [51].

ANTIDEPRESSANTS IN THE TREATMENT OF COMORBID DEPRESSIVE AND ALCOHOL DISORDERS

In principle, the characteristics of the ideal medication for treating alcohol dependence with co-morbid psychiatric illness should include: relief of the psychiatric symptoms, decrease of alcohol use and prevention of relapse, low abuse liability, convenient dose administration to enhance medication adherence, good tolerability and a favorable side-effect profile [52].

Unfortunately, to date, the vast majority of placebo-controlled trials regarding the effectiveness of antidepressants in the treatment of depression excluded individuals with concurrent substance abuse disorders [11, 23]. Furthermore, a number of methodological issues, such as the definition of mood disorder (major depression vs. dysthymia), definition of the alcohol-related disorder (abuse vs. dependence), inclusion of either abstinent or non-abstinent alcoholics in the studies, and their enrollment from outpatient or outpatient settings, complicate the interpretation of data obtained from studies on the treatment of comorbidity [42, 53]. As a result, this heterogeneity makes comparisons between clinical trials awkward and generalization of the findings is limited and uncertain. The clinician is further perplexed by the fact that clinical trials particularly of the '70s and '80s failed to encourage the use of antidepressants for treating depressed alcoholics [54, 55]. These studies, however, were problematic for a number of reasons, such as failure to satisfactorily define the depressive episode, to monitor treatment compliance and to administer adequate doses of the antidepressant [54, 55].

Tricyclic Antidepressants (TCAs)

From the early '90s, TCAs were tried for the treatment of co-occurring depression and alcohol disorders in a number of double-blind placebo-controlled studies. McGrath et al. studied imipramine vs. placebo in 69 outpatient alcoholics with primary depression [56]. The mean daily dosage of imipramine was 260mg and the observation period 12 weeks. Imipramine was superior to placebo in the treatment of depressive symptoms but no overall effect on drinking outcome was observed. Mason et al. conducted another controlled study with desipramine in a sample of 71 alcoholics, 28 of whom had major depression secondary to alcoholism [57]. The mean daily dose was 200mg desipramine for a trial period of 24 weeks. Desipramine was found to be superior to placebo in terms of reduction of depressive symptoms as well as of time to relapse. Of interest, desipramine failed to prevent relapse to drinking in non-depressed alcoholics, which is consistent with earlier studies showing no benefit from TCAs in alcoholics without depressive psychopathology [54, 55].

Selective Serotonin Reuptake Inhibitors (SSRIs)

Given that central nervous system serotonergic dysfunction has been implicated both in alcohol dependence and depression, SSRIs were of particular interest as potential therapeutic agents in the population of depressed alcoholics [11, 42, 58]. Based on their safety, their tolerability and their favorable side-effect profile, investigators have been encouraged to use these medications [42].

Cornelius et al. examined the efficacy of fluoxetine in a placebo-controlled study of 51 alcoholics with severe depression [59]. All patients were initially hospitalized; 90% of them reported suicidal ideation and 35% were admitted following a suicide attempt. Patients received 20-40mg/d of fluoxetine or placebo for a period of 12 weeks. Results showed a significant effect favoring fluoxetine over placebo on depressive symptomatology, as well as significantly greater reductions on most measures of alcohol use. In another study of 101 outpatient alcoholics, the majority of whom (86%) reported mild to moderate depressive symptoms, fluoxetine, compared with placebo, significantly reduced depressive symptoms in individuals with major depression, but was ineffective in the majority of non-depressed patients. Furthermore, fluoxetine had no significant effect on the level of alcohol consumption [60].

Sertraline has been also evaluated in several clinical trials since 1998, with mixed results. In Roy's study, comprising 36 inpatient alcoholics with secondary depression, sertraline (100mg/d) had a more favorable effect than placebo in terms of depression outcome. However, drinking outcome was not reported because all except one participant remained abstinent over the 6-week trial [61]. Petinatti et al. examined the effectiveness of 200mg/day sertraline vs. placebo for 14 weeks in a sample of 100 alcoholics with or without a lifetime diagnosis of comorbid depression [62]. Sertraline was superior to placebo only in patients without lifetime depression regarding alcohol use outcome but had no effect on the outcome of depression. In another trial, 82 subjects with depression and alcohol dependence were randomly assigned to 12 weeks of either 200mg/d sertraline or placebo [63]. Sertraline had an advantage over placebo in reducing depressive symptoms only among female subjects. Given that alcohol-dependent women are more likely than men to suffer from symptoms of depression, the significance of sex in terms of response to antidepressants merits further exploration. In this study, those who received the active medication had fewer drinks per drinking day than subjects who received placebo, but no other differences on drinking outcomes were reported between the two groups [63]. Finally, in a recent well-designed, large, placebo-controlled study of 328 patients with comorbid major depression and alcohol dependence, sertraline (maximum daily dose 200mg/d for a period of 10 weeks) did not prove to be more effective than placebo in reducing depressive symptoms or drinking behavior [64]. The high rate of response within the placebo group may explain these findings.

Nefazodone is a newer serotoninergic antidepressant that acts mainly as an antagonist at the 5-HT$_2$ receptor. There are two controlled clinical trials that used nefazodone in order to treat depressed alcoholics, but their results are contradictory. In the first study by Roy-Byrne et al., up to 500mg/d of nefazodone were given to 64 alcoholics with primary depression for a period of 12 weeks [65]. Nefazodone-treated patients had a more marked reduction of depressive symptoms than those taking placebo, but no significant reduction of alcohol intake was recorded. In a more recent trial, 41 alcoholics with primary depression were randomized to nefazodone (up to 600mg/d for 10 weeks) or placebo, in addition to supportive psychotherapy. Although the nefazodone group showed greater reductions in depressive and anxiety symptoms, the effects did not reach statistical significance. Nonetheless, nefazodone-treated subjects showed a significantly greater reduction in heavy drinking days and in total drinks compared with the placebo-treated subjects [66].

Serotonin and Norepinephrine Reuptake Inhibitors (SNRIs)

Venlafaxine, a serotonin and norepinephrine reuptake inhibitor, was tried in three open-label studies with a small number of patients. Results suggest that it could be effective and well-tolerated for the treatment of patients with comorbid substance abuse and depression [67, 68]. In a Spanish open-label study, without placebo, the effectiveness of venlafaxine was evaluated in 90 alcoholics with major depression [68]. The mean daily dose of venlafaxine was 112mg/d and the observation period 24 weeks. Findings indicated that treatment with venlafaxine was significantly associated with an improvement of the depressive symptoms and alcohol use severity. Furthermore, venlafaxine was well-tolerated by the alcoholics.

Noradrenergic and Specific Serotonergic Antidepressants (NaSSA)

Mirtazapine, a noradrenergic and specific serotonergic antidepressant agent, has been recently used in the treatment of alcohol-dependent individuals undergoing alcohol detoxification. Mirtazapine combined with short-term psychotherapy proved to be efficacious in reducing symptoms of depression and anxiety, thus helping the detoxification process by minimizing physical and psychological discomfort [69].

The 35 patients who were given a combined treatment of psychotherapy and mirtazapine after the first week of alcohol detoxification displayed a significantly better outcome on all clinical measures of mood disturbance than the control group by the end of this 4-week study. It is noteworthy that this improvement was rapid and evident by the end of the first week of mirtazapine administration [69]. In another study by the same group, mirtazapine was also shown to be superior to venlafaxine in the treatment of collateral psycho-pathology during alcohol detoxification [70].

In another open-label 8-week study without a control group, 148 alcoholics with a current depressive episode were treated with mirtazapine (up to 45mg/d); mirtazapine was associated with improvement of mood, decrease of anxiety, and reduction of craving for alcohol [71].

In a more recent uncontrolled trial, mirtazapine and amitriptyline were evaluated in terms of effectiveness and tolerability for the treatment of 44 alcoholics with comorbid depression [72].

Patients were randomized to mirtazapine (mean dose 45mg/d) or amitriptyline (mean dose 125mg/d) for a period of 8 weeks. Both drugs resulted in equivalent reductions of depression and alcohol craving scores, with no statistically significant differences between treatment groups at any assessment point or at endpoint. However, mirtazapine was reported to have a more favorable safety profile than amitriptyline.

Consequently, mirtazapine might have certain advantages over other antidepressants for the management of alcohol craving and depressive symptoms in cases of comorbidity. Larger, placebo-controlled, and follow-up studies are needed to confirm this observation.

OVERVIEW OF EFFICACY OF ANTIDEPRESSANTS IN THE TREATMENT OF COMORBID DEPRESSIVE AND ALCOHOL DISORDERS

Nunes and Levin recently published a meta-analysis of studies on treatment of comorbid depression and substance use disorders with antidepressant medications. The analysis included 14 placebo-controlled trials with a total of 848 subjects [73]. Five studies used TCAs, seven SSRIs and two other antidepressants. Although there was a large variation of efficacy, the authors concluded that antidepressant agents had an overall modest beneficial effect on depressive symptoms and a small effect in decreasing drug and alcohol use. In their meta-analysis, a high placebo response rate was the single best predictor of a non-significant effect of antidepressant treatment. According to their findings, efficacy of antidepressants was more robust in the case of alcohol-dependent compared with drug-dependent individuals. Even if studies using TCAs yielded more positive results than those using SSRIs, the authors suggested that SSRIs should be the first-line medications for depression in the case of drug and alcohol dependence, due to their better tolerability and lower toxicity compared with TCAs.

In another review, Pettinati and colleagues based on data from 8 well-controlled trials using TCAs and serotoninergic antidepressants, conducted over a decade (1994-2004), concluded that treatment of depressed alcoholics provided significant relief from depressive symptoms in 6 out of 8 studies, but had relatively little impact (only 3 out of 8 studies) on reducing heavy drinking in this population [23]. Likewise, the review by Torrens et al. [74] which included 9 clinical trials (some of them with a small sample size) using TCAs, SSRIs, and nefazodone, showed an overall significant improvement on measures of depression in patients receiving antidepressant medications compared with the placebo-treated groups. SSRIs were not superior to other antidepressants in the management of psychopathology. Moreover, the usefulness of antidepressants in achieving a better drinking outcome was not supported; whenever an improvement was recorded, that effect appeared to be related to the decrease of depressive symptoms. According to the same review, use of antidepressants (either SSRIs or other antidepressants) for the treatment of alcoholics without comorbid depression had no significant effect on alcohol use.

Several issues regarding the selective efficacy of antidepressants in the treatment of patients meeting criteria for specific subtypes of alcohol dependence may be of clinical importance. To this end, two studies tried to investigate whether distinct subgroups of alcoholics respond differently to antidepressants. Contrary to prediction, results suggested that patients with the putatively more severe subtype of alcoholism, i.e., with earlier onset of alcohol dependence, with a family history of alcohol-related disorders, and more psychopathology or sociopathy (Type B or Type 2 of alcoholism), had a less favorable drinking outcome if treated with SSRIs [6, 42, 75, 76]. Further research is needed in order to examine the possible influence of alcoholic typology on drinking outcome in depressed alcoholics.

Another clinically significant concern is the possible influence of sex on treatment outcome. Women seem to be at a higher risk than men for co-occurring depression and alcohol dependence and therefore represent a large proportion of the participants in various studies [2, 77, 78]. In the Moak et al. study, female alcoholics treated with sertraline improved more than males in terms of depressive symptomatology, but no sex differences were detected in drinking outcomes [65]. Two more clinical trials suggest that male alcoholics without symptoms of depression have a better drinking outcome than women when treated with an SSRI [62, 79]. More studies are required in order to investigate the possibility that sex may be a factor influencing outcome in pharmacological studies of patients with comorbid depression and alcoholism.

SELECTING AN ANTIDEPRESSANT

From a clinical standpoint, management of comorbid alcohol abuse and depression can be distinguished into three phases. The first acute phase aims at the patient's engagement in therapy, detoxification from alcohol, relief from physical or psychological discomfort, and treatment of depression. This phase may require an extended period of time if there is little commitment to abstinence. The second phase, the continuation phase, is focused mainly on supporting sobriety but also to further reduce mood symptoms. The last phase is the maintenance phase, which intends to prevent relapse of both conditions [80, 81].

During the first phase of detoxification, various options exist for the effective treatment of symptoms of alcohol withdrawal. Long-acting benzodiazepines are usually the preferred medications. Thereafter, as symptoms of depression and anxiety may substantially subside during the weeks following cessation of drinking, a careful evaluation of psycho-pathology should be done before starting any antidepressant medication.

Available evidence suggests that antidepressant treatment can improve depressive symptomatology in alcohol-dependent individuals with comorbid depression. Chances for response are maximized by sobriety, adherence to treatment, and careful monitoring of the patient [11]. An increasing number of pharmacological agents are nowadays available for the treatment of depression in this context [23, 42]. Besides the desired antidepressant effect, a favorable side effect profile, a low lethality potential on overdose and a low potential for adverse interactions with other drugs or alcohol are indispensable [82]. Although both TCAs and SSRIs will help a significant proportion of alcohol-dependent patients with depression, SSRIs must be the first choice due to their better tolerability and their safety in overdose [23]. Moreover, SSRIs are advantageous as for their action on impulsivity, compulsivity, anxiety or irritability, behaviors closely related to alcohol abuse [11, 83]. Results from clinical studies do not support that individual patients preferably respond better to one SSRI over another. In case of failure of the first SSRI tried, at least one within-class switch is recommended before considering another option [11]. Alternative options include mirtazapine and venlafaxine.

Alcohol's interactions with medications are a crucial issue in the field of treatment of alcoholism with comorbidity. A large proportion of alcoholics take a number of other medications, such as antidepressants, sedatives, antipsychotics, etc. It is estimated that alcohol-medications interactions may be a factor in at least 25% of all emergency room admissions [84]. Alcohol-medications interactions can be distinguished into two categories: pharmacokinetic interactions, where alcohol directly interferes with the normal metabolism of the medication through metabolizing enzyme inhibition or activation, and pharmacodynamic interaction, which refers to the additive effects of alcohol and medications [85]. In this second type of interaction, which most often occurs in the central nervous system, alcohol alters the effects of medication without changing its concentration in the blood. Interestingly, pharmacodynamic interaction can take place even with intermittent alcohol consumption or after a single dose of a drink [85].

From the various types of antidepressants, TCAs exhibit the most serious interactions with alcohol. Alcohol increases TCAs' sedative effects through pharmacodynamic interactions [85]. In addition, alcohol use can cause pharmacokinetic interactions with these compounds, resulting in increased blood levels of antidepressants or increased bioavailability, which in turn can lead to convulsions and cardiac arrhythmias. Conversely, SSRIs have no serious interactions when consumed with moderate alcohol quantities, presenting the best safety profile of all antidepressants [11, 73, 85]. From the rest of antidepressants, monoaminoxidase inhibitors (MAOI) can induce a dangerous rise of blood pressure when taken together with tyramine, which is found in some beers or in red wine; as little as one standard drink may expose to the risk that such an interaction will occur [85]. Finally, nefazodone and trazodone, as well as mirtazapine, may enhance sedation when consumed with alcohol [85].

In a recent Finnish study, postmortem toxicology data were analyzed in order to establish more precisely fatal toxicity indices for the newer antidepressants and to evaluate their interaction with alcohol [86]. It came out that more than half of the 284 cases of fatal poisoning involved antidepressants and alcohol interaction. The authors concluded that SSRIs appear to have a lower risk of fatal poisoning when taken alone or in combination with alcohol, whereas antidepressants such as venlafaxine, mianserin, moclobemide and mirtazapine are associated with an elevated risk, having an additive or synergistic interaction with alcohol [86]. As alcohol abusing patients with concurrent depressive episodes form a high risk population for taking higher than prescribed doses of their medications, knowledge of alcohol-medications interactions is crucial for the choice of antidepressant.

MOOD STABILIZERS AND ANTICONVULSANTS IN THE TREATMENT OF DEPRESSED ALCOHOLICS

Investigations on the efficacy of lithium in the treatment of alcoholism began in the '70s with mixed results [87, 88, 89]. More recent and larger clinical trials failed to confirm that lithium is effective for the treatment of individuals with alcohol use disorders. In 1989, Dorus et al. administered lithium to 457 outpatient alcoholic men, with or without depressive symptoms, in a well-designed double-blind, placebo-controlled 52-week study [90]. Lithium treatment was not effective regarding drinking outcome measures, either in depressed or non-depressed alcoholics, and did not affect severity of depressive symptoms. In another 6-month, double-bind, placebo-controlled study of 156 alcoholics, no differences were detected between lithium carbonate, buspirone or placebo in reducing alcohol use [91]. Geller and colleagues evaluated the efficacy of lithium treatment in a small, randomized, placebo-controlled, 6-week trial of 21 adolescents with bipolar disorders and secondary substance dependence; concurrent abuse of alcohol and marijuana was the most frequent abuse [92]. Lithium was an effective treatment for both alcohol abuse and bipolar disorder in this group of adolescents; yet, the results need replication with a longer follow-up period during the maintenance phase. Finally, in a review of both controlled and uncontrolled studies of lithium treatment for alcoholism, the authors concluded that lithium did not demonstrate efficacy in either depressed or non-depressed alcoholics [93]. Moreover, the safety profile of lithium is probably incompatible with its use in an outpatient basis for the treatment of alcohol dependence.

Despite the frequent co-occurrence of bipolar disorder and alcoholism, there is a lack of evidence-based effective pharmacological treatment for patients with comorbid alcohol abuse and bipolar disorder. This is due to the systematic exclusion of bipolar patients from clinical trials. However, a number of clinical trials suggest the usefulness of certain anticonvulsants such as carbamazepine, valproic acid, gabapentin, and topiramate in the treatment of withdrawal symptoms and the prevention of relapse to alcohol use [94, 95, 96].

In a recent 24-week, double-blind, placebo-controlled study, the efficacy of valproate in decreasing alcohol use and stabilizing mood symptoms in 59 alcoholics with bipolar I disorder was evaluated. All participants were on a standard treatment consisting of lithium and weekly individual counseling. Valproate was shown to decrease heavy drinking among bipolar alcoholics beyond its effect on mood, as manic and depressive symptoms improved equally in both groups [97]. In another open-label, naturalistic trial with no blind, 20 alcoholics with comorbid mood disorder, mainly of the bipolar I or II type, were treated with divalproex at a mean dose of 1075mg/day. Significant improvement in mood and alcohol-related outcome measures was reported by the majority of patients. In 13 of them divalproex sodium was safely combined with other psychiatric medications, mainly antidepressants [98].

Lamotrigine was tried in another 12-week open-label study without a control group comprising 28 outpatients with comorbid alcoholism and bipolar disorder. Lamotrigine was used as adjunctive therapy to other medications, such as lithium, gabapentin or atypical antipsychotics. Lamotrigine was shown to improve mood symptoms in bipolar alcoholics, to decrease alcohol consumption and craving for alcohol, and was well tolerated [99]. In overall, the use of newer anticonvulsants, which have lower toxicity, fewer side effects, lower interaction with alcohol and no potential for abuse, is emerging as a promising treatment in the context of comorbidity of alcoholism and affective disorders [94, 95, 100].

CONCLUSION

Alcohol abuse/dependence and affective disorders frequently co-exist and have a considerable impact on the prognosis and treatment of each one of these conditions. Recently, there has been an increased interest in the treatment of individuals suffering from both disorders. Findings reported in the present article are inconclusive but quite promising. Thus, TCAs and SSRIs appear to be efficient for the treatment of depressive symptoms in cases of comorbidity but less effective for the reduction of alcohol consumption. Needless to mention that safety and side-effect profile of the medications used should be a priority in the treatment of individuals who misuse alcohol. Also, they underscore the need for better designed pharmacological studies that target psychiatric comorbidity; future trials should also evaluate combinations of medications. In general, efforts should be made to effectively integrate pharmacotherapies with psychotherapeutic approaches. Pharmacotherapy combined with psychotherapeutic and psychosocial interventions targeting both disorders may be a much more effective approach to the management of comorbidity in depressed alcoholics.

REFERENCES

[1]   Schuckit MA, Tipp JE, Bucholz KK, Nurnberger JI, Hesselbrock VM, Crowe RR, Kramer J: The lifetime rates of three major mood disorders and four anxiety disorders in alcoholics and controls. *Addiction* 1997; 92(10):1289-1304.

[2]   Kessler RC, Crum RM, Warner LA, Nelson CB, Schulenberg J, Anthony JC: Lifetime co-occurrence of DSM-III-R alcohol abuse and dependence with other psychiatric disorders in the National Comorbidity Survey. *Arch. Gen. Psychiatry* 1997; 54:313-321.

[3]   Grant BF, Harford TC: Comorbidity between DSM-IV alcohol use disorders and major depression: results of a national survey. *Drug Alcohol Depend.* 1995; 39:197-206.

[4]   Hasin DS, Stinson FS, Ogburn E, Grant BF: Prevalence, correlates, disability, and comorbidity of DSM-IV alcohol abuse and dependence in the United States: results from the National Epidemiologic Survey on Alcohol and Related Conditions. *Arch. Gen. Psychiatry* 2007; 64:830-842.

[5]   Hasin DS, Goodwin RD, Stinson FS, Grant BF: Epidemiology of major depressive disorder: results from the National Epidemiologic Survey on Alcoholism and Related Conditions. *Arch. Gen. Psychiatry* 2005; 62:1097-1106.

[6]   Myrick H, Cluver J, Swavely S, Peters H: Diagnosis and treatment of co-occurring affective disorders and substance use disorders. *Psychiatr. Clin. North Am.* 2004; 27:649-659.

[7]   Merikangas KR, Gelernter CS: Comorbidity for alcoholism and depression. *Psychiatr. Clin. North Am.* 1990; 13:613-632.

[8]   Lynskey MT: The comorbidity of alcohol dependence and affective disorders: treatment implications. *Drug Alcohol Depend.* 1998; 52:201-209.

[9]   Hasin DS, Wei-Yuan T, Endicott J: The effects of major depression on alcoholism: five-years course. *Am. J. Addict.* 1996; 5:144-155.

[10] Curran GM, Flynn HA, Kirchner J: Depression after alcohol treatment as a risk factor for relapse among male veterans. *J. Subst. Abuse Treat.* 2000; 19:259-265.

[11] Thase ME, Salloum IM, Cornelius JD: Comorbid alcoholism and depression: treatment issues. *J. Clin.. Psychiatry* 2001; 62(suppl 20):32-41.

[12] Fortney JC, Booth BM, Curran GM: Do patients with alcohol dependence use more services? A comparative analysis with other chronic disorders. *Alcohol. Clin. Exp. Res.* 1999; 23:127-133.

[13] Grant BF, Hasin DS: Suicidal ideation among the United States drinking population: results from the National Longitudinal Alcohol Epidemiologic Survey. *J. Stud. Alcohol.* 1999; 60:422-429.

[14] Wang JL, El-Guebaly NA: Sociodemographic factors associated with comorbid major depressive episodes and alcohol dependence in the general population. *Can. J. Psychiatry* 2004; 49:37-44.

[15] Regier DA, Farmer ME, Rae DE, Locke BZ, Keith EJ, Judd LL, Goodwin EK: Comorbidity of mental disorders with alcohol and other drug abuse: results from the Epidemiologic Catchment Area (ECA) study. *JAMA* 1990; 264:2511-2518.

[16] Schuckit MA, Tipp JE, Bergman M, Reich W, Hesselbrock VM, Smith TL: Comparison of induced and independent major depressive disorders in 2,945 alcoholics. *Am. J. Psychiatry* 1997; 154:948-957.

[17] Grant BF, Stinson FS, Dawson DA, Chou SP, Dufour MC, Compton W, Pickering RP, Kaplan K: Prevalence and co-occurrence of substance use disorders and independent mood and anxiety disorders: results from the National Epidemiologic Survey on Alcohol and Related Conditions. *Arch. Gen. Psychiatry* 2004; 61:807-816.

[18] Ross HE: DSM-III-R alcohol use and dependence and psychiatric comorbidity in Ontario: results from the mental health supplement to the Ontario Health Survey. *Drug Alcohol Depend.* 1995; 39:111-128.

[19] Grant BF, Hasin DS, Dawson DA: The relationship between DSM-IV alcohol use disorders and DSM-IV major depression: examination of the primary-secondary distinction in a general population sample. *J. Affect. Disord.* 1996; 38:113-128.

[20] Burns L, Teesson M: Alcohol use disorders comorbid with anxiety, depression and drug use disorders. Findings from the Australian National Survey of Mental Health and Well Being. *Drug Alcohol Depend.* 2002; 68:299-307.

[21] Schuckit MA: The clinical implications of primary diagnostic groups among alcoholics. *Arch. Gen. Psychiatry* 1985; 42:1043-1049.

[22] American Psychiatric Association: Diagnostic and Statistical Manual of Mental Disorders (4th ed). Washington, DC, American Psychiatric Press, 1994.

[23] Pettinati HM: Antidepressant treatment of co-occuring depression and alcohol dependence. *Biol. Psychiatry* 2004; 56:785-792.

[24] Ramsey SE, Kahler CW, Read JP, Stuart GL, Brown RA: Discriminating between substance-induced and independent depressive episodes in alcohol dependent patients. *J. Stud. Alcohol.* 2004; 65:672-676.

[25] Schuckit MA, Smith TL, Danko GP, Pierson J, Trim R, Nurnberger JI, Kramer J, Kuperman S, Bierut LJ, Hesselbrock V: A comparison of factors associated with substance-induced versus independent depressions. *J. Stud. Alcohol Drugs* 2007; 68:805-812.

[26] Schuckit MA: Alcohol and depression: a clinical perspective. *Acta Psychiatr. Scand.* 1994: 377(Suppl):28-32.

[27] Hesselbrock MN, Hesselbrock VM, Segal B, Schuckit MA, Bucholz K: Ethnicity and psychiatric comorbidity among alcohol-dependent persons who receive inpatient treatment: African Americans, Alaska natives, Caucasians, and Hispanics. *Alcohol. Clin. Exp. Res.* 2003; 27:1368-73.

[28] Powel BJ, Read MR, Penick EC, Miller NS, Bingham SF: Primary and secondary depression in alcoholic men: an important distinction. *J. Clin. Psychiatry* 1987; 48:98-101.

[29] Hasegawa K, Mukasa N, Nakazawa Y, Kodama H, Nakamura K: Primary and secondary depression in alcoholism: clinical features and family history. *Drug Alcohol Depend.* 1991; 27:275-281.

[30] Schuckit MA: Drug and Alcohol Abuse: a clinical guide to diagnosis and treatment (5th ed), New York: Springer; 2000, pp.60.

[31] Caron C, Rutter M: Comorbidity in child psychopathology: concepts, issues and research strategies. *J. Child Psychol. Psychiatry* 1991; 32:1063-1080.

[32] Chutuape MAD, De Wit H: Preferences of ethanol and diazepam in anxious individuals: an evaluation of the self-medication hypothesis. *Psychopharmacology* 1995; 121:91-103.

[33] Kuo PH, Gardner CO, Kendler KS, Prescot CA: The temporal relationship of the onsets of alcohol dependence and major depression: using a genetically informative study design. *Psychol. Med.* 2006; 36:1153-1162.

[34] Abraham HD, Fava M: Order of onset of substance abuse and depression in a sample of depression in a sample of depressed outpatients. *Compr. Psychiatry* 1999; 40:44-50.

[35] Crum RM, Storr CL, Chan YF: Depression syndromes with risk of alcohol dependence in adulthood: a latent class analysis. *Drug Alcohol Depend.* 2005; 79:71-81.

[36] Nurnberger JI, Foroud T, Flury L, Meyer ET, Wiegand R: Is there a genetic relationship between alcoholism and depression? *Alcohol Res. Health* 2002; 26(3):233-240.

[37] Tambs K, Harris JR, Magnus P: Genetic and environmental contributions to the correlation between alcohol consumption and symptoms of anxiety and depression: results from a bivariate analysis of Norwegian twin data. *Behav. Genet.* 1997; 27:241-250.

[38] Edenberg HJ: The Collaborative Study on the Genetics of Alcoholism: an update. *Alcohol Res. Health* 2002; 26:214-218.

[39] Nurnberger JI, Foroud T, Flury L, Su J, Meyer ET, Hu K, Crowe R, Edenberg H, Goate A, Bierut L, Reich T, Schuckit M, Reich W: Evidence for a locus on chromosome 1 that influences vulnerability to alcoholism and affective disorders. *Am. J. Psychiatry* 2001; 158(5): 718-724.

[40] Litten RZ, Allen JP: Advances in development of medications for alcoholism treatment. *Psychopharmacology* 1998; 139:20-23.

[41] Weiss RD: Pharmacotherapy for co-occuring mood and substance use disorders, in Intregrated Treatment for Mood and Substance Use Disorders. Edited by Westrmeyer JJ, Weiss RD, Ziedonis DM. Baltimore, The John Hopkins University Press 2001, pp. 122-139.

[42] Le Fauve CE, Litten RZ, Randall CR, Moak DH, Salloum IM, Green AI : Pharmacological treatment of alcohol abuse/dependence with psychiatric comorbidity. *Alcohol. Clin.. Exp. Res.* 2004; 28:302-312.

[43] Galanter M, Kleber HD: Textbook of substance abuse treatment, 2nd ed. Washington, DC, American Psychiatric Press 1999, pp.157-158.

[44] Goldsmith RJ, Ries RK: Substance-induced mental disorders, in Principles of Addiction Medicine (3rd ed.). Edited by Graham AW, Schulz TK, Mayo-Smith MF, Ries RK, Wilford BB. Chevy Chase, American Society of Addiction Medicine, pp.1263-1276.

[45] Thevos AK, Johnston AL, Latham PK, Randall CL, Adinoff B, Malcolm R: Symptoms of anxiety in inpatient alcoholics with and without DSM-III-R anxiety diagnoses. *Alcohol. Clin. Exp. Res.* 1991; 15:102-105.

[46] Brown SA, Inaba RK, Gillin JC, Schuckit MA, Stewart MA, Irwin MR: Alcoholism and affective disorder: clinical course of depressive symptoms. *Am. J. Psychiatry* 1995; 152(1):45-52.

[47] Liappas J, Paparrigopoulos T, Tzavellas E, Christodoulou G: Impact of alcohol detoxification on anxiety and depressive symptoms. *Drug Alcohol Depend.* 2002; 68:215-220.

[48] Barlow DH, Lehman CL: Advances in the psychosocial treatment of anxiety disorders: implications for national health care. *Arch. Gen. Psychiatry* 1996; 53:727-735.

[49] Anton RF, Moak DH, Waid LR, Latham PK, Malcolm RJ, Dias JK: Naltrexone and cognitive behavioral therapy for the treatment of outpatient alcoholics: results of a placebo-controlled trial. *Am. J. Psychiatry* 1999; 156:1758-1764.

[50] Brown RA, Evans M, Miller IW, Burgess ES, Mueller TI: Cognitive-behavioral treatment for depression in alcoholism. *J. Consult. Clin. Psychol.* 1997; 65:715-726.

[51] Group MATCH Research Group: Matching alcoholism treatments to client heterogeneity: treatment main effects and matching effects on drinking during treatment. *J. Stud.. Alcohol.* 1998; 59:631-639.

[52] Golstein BI, Diamantouros A, Schaffer A, Naranjo C: Pharmacotherapy of alcoholism with co-morbid psychiatric disorders. *Drugs* 2006; 66(9):1229-1237.

[53] Ostacher MJ: Comorbid alcohol and substance abuse dependence in depression: impact on the outcome of antidepressant treatment. *Psychiatr. Clin. North Am.* 2007; 30:69-76.

[54] Ciraulo DA, Jaffe JH: Tricyclic antidepressants in the treatment of depression associated with alcoholism. *J. Clin. Psychopharmacol.* 1981; 1(3):146-150.

[55] Liskow BI, Goodwin DW: Pharmacological treatment of alcohol intoxication, withdrawal and dependence: a critical review. *J. Stud. Alcohol.* 1987; 48:356-370.

[56] McGrath PJ, Nunes EV, Stewart JW, Goldman D, Agosti V, Ocepek-Welikson K, Quitkin FM: Imipramine treatment of alcoholics with primary depression: a placebo-controlled clinical trial. *Arch. Gen. Psychiatry* 1996; 53:232-240.

[57] Mason BJ, Kocsis JH, Ritvo EC, Cutler RB: A double-blind, placebo-controlled trial of desipramine for primary alcohol dependence stratified on the presence or absence of major depression. *JAMA* 1996; 275:761-767.

[58]   Naranjo CA, Knoke DM: The role of selective serotonin reuptake
        inhibitors in reducing alcohol consumption. *J. Clin. Psychiatry* 2001;
        62(suppl. 20):18-25.

[59]   Cornelius JR, Salloum IM, Ehler JG, Jarrett PJ, Cornelius MD, Perel
        JM, Thase ME, Black A: Fluoxetine in depressed alcoholics: a double-
        blind, placebo-controlled trial. *Arch. Gen. Psychiatry* 1997; 54:700-705.

[60]   Kranzler HR, Burleson JA, Korner P, Del Boca FK, Bohn MJ, Brown J,
        Liebowitz N: Placebo-controlled trial of fluoxetine as an adjunct to
        relapse prevention in alcoholics. *Am. J. Psychiatry* 1995;152:391-397.

[61]   Roy A: Placebo-controlled study of sertraline in depressed recently
        abstinent alcoholics. *Biol. Psychiatry* 1998; 44:633-637.

[62]   Pettinati HM, Volpicelli JR, Luck G, Kranzler HR, Rukstalis MR, Cnaan
        A: Double-blind clinical trial of sertraline treatment for alcohol
        dependence. *J. Clin. Psychopharmacol.* 2001; 21: 143-153.

[63]   Moak DA, Anton RF, Latham PK, Voronin KE, Waid RL, Durazo-
        Arvizu R: Sertraline and cognitive behavioral therapy for depressed
        alcoholics: Results of a placebo- controlled trial. *J. Clin.
        Psychopharmacol.* 2003; 23:553-562.

[64]   Kranzler HR, Mueller T, Cornelius J, Pettinati HM, Moak D, Martin PR,
        Anthenelli R, Brower KJ, O'Malley S, Mason BJ, Hasin D, Keller M:
        Sertraline treatment of co-occuring alcohol dependence and major
        depression. *J. Clin. Psychopharmacol.* 2006; 26:13-20.

[65]   Roy-Byrne PP, Pages KP, Russo JE, Jaffe C, Blume AW, Kingsley E,
        Cowley DS, Ries RK: Nefazodone treatment of major depression in
        alcohol-dependent patients: a double-blind, placebo-controlled trial. *J.
        Clin. Psychopharmacol.* 2000; 20:129-136.

[66]   Hernandez-Avila CA, Modesto-Lowe V, Feinn R, Kranzler HR:
        Nefazodone treatment of comorbid alcohol dependence and major
        depression. *Alcohol. Clin. Exp. Res.* 2004; 28:433-440.

[67]   McDowell DM, Levin FR, Seracini AM, Nunes EV: Venlafaxine
        treatment of cocaine abusers with depressive disorders. *Am. J. Drug
        Alcohol Abuse* 2000; 26:25-31.

[68]   Garcia-Portilla MP, Bascaran MT, Saiz PA, Mateos M, Gonzalez-Quiros
        M, Perez P, Avila JJ, Torres MA, Bombin B, Caso C, Marin R, Prieto R,
        Bobes J: Effectiveness of venlafaxine of alcohol dependence with
        comorbid depression. *Actas Esp. Psiquiatr.* 2005; 33:41-45.

[69]   Liappas J, T.Paparrigopoulos, Malitas P, Tzavellas E, Christodoulou G:
        Mirtazapine improves alcohol detoxification. *J. Psycopharmacol.* 2004;
        18(1):88-93.

[70] Liappas J, Paparrigopoulos T, Tzavellas E, Rabavilas A: Mirtazapine and venlafaxine in the management of collateral psychopathology during alcohol detoxification. *Prog. Neuropsychopharmacol. Biol. Psychiatry* 2005; 29:55-60.

[71] Yoon SJ, Pae CU, Kim DJ, Namkoong K, Lee E, Oh DY, Lee YS, Shin DH, Joeng YC, Kim JH, Choi SB, Hwang IB, Shin YC, Cho SN, Lee HK, Lee CT: Mirtazapine for patients with alcohol dependence and comorbid depressive disorders: a multicentre, open label study. *Prog. Neuropsychopharmacol. Biol. Psychiatry* 2006; 30:1196-1201.

[72] Altintoprak AE, Zorlu N, Coskunol H, Akdeniz F, Kitapcioglu G: Effectiveness and tolerability of mirtazapine and amitriptyline in alcoholic patients with co-morbid depressive disorder: a randomized, double-blind study. *Hum. Psychopharmacol. Clin. Exp.* 2008; 10:313-319.

[73] Nunes EV, Levin FR: Treatment of depression in patients with alcohol or other drug dependence: a meta-analysis. *JAMA* 2004; 291:1887-1896.

[74] Torrens M, Fonseca F, Mateu G, Farre M: Efficacy of antidepressants in substance use disorders with and without comorbid depression. A systematic review and meta-analysis. *Drug Alcohol Depend.* 2005; 78:1-22.

[75] Pettinati H: The use of selective serotonin reuptake inhibitors in treating alcoholic subtypes. *J. Clin. Psychiatry* 2001; 62(suppl 20):26-31.

[76] Kranzler HR, Burleson JA, Brown J, Babor TF: Fluoxetine treatment seems to reduce the beneficial effects of cognitive-behavioral therapy in type B alcoholics. *Alcohol. Clin. Exp. Res.* 1996; 20:1534-1541.

[77] Dixit AR, Crum RM: Prospective study of depression and the risk of heavy alcohol use in women. *Am. J. Psychiatry* 2000; 157:751-758.

[78] Spak L, Spak F, Allebeck P: Alcoholism and depression in a Swedish female population: co-morbidity and risk factors. *Acta Psychiatr. Scand.* 2000; 102:44-51.

[79] Pettinati HM, Dundon WD, Lipkin C: Gender differences in response to sertraline pharmacotherapy in Type A alcohol dependence. *Am. J. Addict.* 2004; 13:236-247.

[80] Salloum IM, Daley DC, Thase ME: Male depression, alcoholism and violence. London, England; Martin Dunitz Ltd; 2000.

[81] Mariani JJ, Levin FR: Pharmacotherapy for alcohol-related disorders: what clinicians should know. *Am. J. Addict.* 2007; 16 (Suppl 1):45-54.

[82] Thase ME, Kupfer DJ: Recent developments in the pharmacotherapy of mood disorders. *J. Consult. Clin. Psychol.* 1996; 64:646-659.

[83] McGrath PJ, Nunes EV, Quitkin FM: Current concepts in the treatment of depression in alcohol-dependent patients. *Psychiatr. Clin. North Am.* 2000; 23:695-711.

[84] Alcohol-Medications Interactions. NIAAA Publications. No 27. 1995.

[85] Weathermon R, Crabb D: Alcohol and medications interactions. *Alcohol Res. Health* 1999; 23:40-54.

[86] Koski A, Vuori E, Ojanpera I: Newer antidepressants: evaluation of fatal toxicity index and interaction with alcohol based on Finnish postmortem data. *Int. J. Legal Med.* 2005; 119:344-8.

[87] Kline NS, Wren JC, Cooper TB, Varga E, Canal O: Evaluation of lithium therapy in chronic and periodic alcoholism. *Am. J. Med. Sci.* 1974; 268:15-22.

[88] Merry J, Reynolds CM, Bailey J, Coppen A: Prophylactic treatment of alcoholism by lithium carbonate: a controlled study. *Lancet* 1976; 1:481-482.

[89] Fawcett J, Clark DC, Aagesen DO, Pisani VD, Tilkin JM, Sellers D, McGuire M, Gibbons RD: A double-blind, placebo-controlled trial of lithium carbonate therapy for alcoholism. *Arch. Gen. Psychiatry* 1987; 44:248-256.

[90] Dorus W, Ostrow D, Anton R, Cushman P, Collins JF, Schaefer M, Charles HL, Desai P, Hayashida M, Malkerneker U, Willenbring M, Fiscella R, Sather M: Lithium treatment of depressed and nondepressed alcoholics. *JAMA* 1989; 262:1646-1652.

[91] Fawcett J, Kravitz HM, McGuire M, Easton M, Ross J, Pisani VD, Fogg LF, Clark D, Whitney M, Kravitz G, Javaid J, Teas G: Pharmacological treatments for alcoholism: revisiting lithium and considering buspirone. *Alcohol Clin. Exp. Res.* 2000; 24:666-674.

[92] Geller B, Cooper TB, Sun K, Zimerman B, Frazier J, Williams M, Heath J: Double blind and placebo controlled study of lithium for adolescent bipolar disorders with secondary substance dependency. *J. Am. Acad. Child Adolesc.* 1998; 37:171-178.

[93] Lejoyeux M, Ades J: Evaluation of lithium treatment in alcoholism. *Alcohol Alcoholism* 1993; 28:273-279.

[94] Frey MA, Salloum IM: Bipolar disorder and comorbid alcoholism: prevalence rates and treatment considerations. *Bipolar Disord.* 2006; 8:677-685.

[95] Myrick H, Brady K, Malcolm R: New developments in the pharmacotherapy of alcohol dependence. *Am. J. Addict.* 2001; 10(suppl):3-15.

[96] Rosenberg J, Salzman C: Update: new uses of lithium and anticonvulsants. *CNS Spectr.* 2007; 12:831-841.

[97] Salloum IM, Cornelius JR, Daley D, Kirisci L, Himmelhoch JM, Thase ME: Efficacy of valproate maintenance in patients with bipolar disorder and alcoholism. *Arch. Gen. Psychiatry* 2005; 62:37-45.

[98] Albanese MJ, Clodfelter RC, Khantzian EJ: Divalproex sodium in substance abusers with mood disorder. *J. Clin. Psychiatry* 2000; 61:916-921.

[99] Rubio G, Lopez-Munoz F, Alamo C: Effects of lamotrigine in patients with bipolar disorder and alcohol dependence. *Bipolar Disord.* 2006; 8:289-293.

[100] Johnson BA: An overview of the development of medications including novel anticonvulsants for the treatment of alcohol dependence. *Expert Opin. Pharmacother.* 2004; 5:1943-1955.

INDEX